The Rehabilitation of People With Traumatic Brain Injury

Buck H. Woo, PhD
Editor

Assistant Professor of Rehabilitation Medicine
Boston University School of Medicine

Neuropsychologist
Neurological and Cognitive Rehabilitation Programs
Boston Medical Center

Shanker Nesathurai, MD, FRCP(C)
Editor

Chairman *ad interim* of Rehabilitation Medicine
Associate Professor of Rehabilitation Medicine
Boston University School of Medicine

Chief of Rehabilitation Services
Boston Medical Center

Published 2000
ISBN # 0-632-04517-5
Library of Congress # pending publication
©2000 by Boston Medical Center
www.bumc.bu.edu/rehab
www.bmc.org/rehab

Blackwell Science, Inc.

b

Blackwell
Science

©2000 by Boston Medical Center

Blackwell Science, Inc.

Editorial Offices:
Commerce Place, 350 Main Street, Malden, Massachusetts 02148, USA
Osney Mead, Oxford OX2 0EL, England
25 John Street, London WC1N 2BL, England
23 Ainslie Place, Edinburgh EH3 6AJ, Scotland
54 University Street, Carlton, Victoria 3053, Australia
Other Editorial Offices:
Blackwell Wissenschafts-Verlag GmbH, Kurfürstendamn 57, 10707 Berlin, Germany
Blackwell Science KK, MG Kodenmacho Building, 7-10 Kodenmacho Nihombashi,
Chuo-ku, Tokyo 104, Japan

Distributors:

USA
    Blackwell Science, Inc.
    Commerce Place
    350 Main Street
    Malden, Massachusetts 02148
    (Telephone orders: 800-215-1000 or
    781-388-8250; fax orders: 781-388-8270)

Australia
    Blackwell Science Pty, Ltd.
    54 University Street
    Carlton, Victoria 3053
    (Telephone orders: 03-9347-0300;
    fax orders: 03-9349-3016)

Canada
    Login Brothers Book Company
    324 Saulteaux Crescent
    Winnipeg, Manitoba, R3J 3T2
    (Telephone orders: 204-837-2987)

Outside North America and Australia
    Blackwell Science, Ltd.
    c/o Marston Book Services, Ltd.
    P.O. Box 269
    Abingdon
    Oxon OX14 4YN
    England
    (Telephone orders: 44-01235-465500;
    fax orders: 44-01235-465555)

This book is dedicated to the residents in the physical medicine and rehabilitation program at Boston Medical Center.

Table of Contents

Acknowledgments

The development and distribution of this monograph is supported by an unrestricted grant from Athena Neurosciences, a division of Elan Pharmaceuticals, Inc., to the Department of Rehabilitation Medicine at the Boston University School of Medicine. The Department is grateful for the support of Michelle Finnegan-Saunders, Stacey Garson and Marianne Lambertson for facilitating the project. This monograph is being distributed without cost to junior rehabilitation medicine residents as part of Boston University School of Medicine's mission of disseminating knowledge and educating health-care professionals. Additional copies are available at a nominal cost by contacting the publisher (see page 127).

The Department of Rehabilitation Medicine is the recipient of a National Institute on Disability and Rehabilitation Research grant (H133N950014-99A).

The authors are grateful to the following clinicians for reviewing the manuscript and providing insightful criticisms: Drs. Kathleen Abbott, Chumbo Cai, Daniel Carney, Maturin Finch, Mel B. Glenn, Allan Meyers, and Radha Vijayakumar.

We would also like to express our gratitude to Scott Edwards, Patricia Regan, and Marjorie Scott for their editorial assistance; Jason Laramie for the original artwork in this monograph; Lisa Gollihue for her typesetting and design; and John Bertolami of the Boston Medical Center Outpatient Pharmacy for his assistance with drug pricing.

Although the contributors are grateful for the support provided by their respective institutions, the opinions and comments expressed in this monograph are those of the authors. The opinions given are not endorsed by any organization, agency or reviewer. We would also like to thank Dr. Joel Myklebust for his support.

Most of all, we would like to thank our wives, Lygia Soares and Nancy Nesathurai, for their patience and support throughout this project's preparation.

Contributors

Boston Medical Center

Anantha Kamath, MD
Senior Resident in Rehabilitation Medicine

Mark Kaplan, MD
Assistant Professor of Rehabilitation Medicine
Boston University School of Medicine

Shanker Nesathurai, MD, FRCP(C)
Associate Professor of Rehabilitation Medicine
Boston University School of Medicine

Joe I. Ordia, MD, FACS
Professor of Neurological Surgery
Boston University School of Medicine

Emilia Semenov, MD
Senior Resident in Rehabilitation Medicine

Michael Stillman
Medical Student
Boston University School of Medicine

Georgia Thoidis, MA, MPH
Medical Student
Boston University School of Medicine

Steven Williams, MD
Assistant Professor of Rehabilitation Medicine
Boston University School of Medicine

Buck H. Woo, PhD
Assistant Professor of Rehabilitation Medicine
Boston University School of Medicine

Harvard Medical School

David Burke, MD, MA
Director of Brain Injury Programs
Assistant Professor of Rehabilitation Medicine

Northwestern University Medical School

Steven Nussbaum, MD
Assistant Professor of Rehabilitation Medicine
Rehabilitation Institute of Chicago

University of New Hampshire

Lygia Soares, PhD
Adjunct Assistant Professor of Communication Disorders

University of Massachusetts Medical School

Elizabeth Roaf, MD
Assistant Professor of Orthopedics and
Physical Rehabiliation
Medical Director, Fairlawn Rehabilitation Hospital

University of Southern California

Douglas E. Garland, MD
Clinical Professor of Surgery

Mentor Community Brain Injury Program

Troy Scherer
Clinical Coordinator

Overview

Buck H. Woo, PhD
Shanker Nesathurai, MD, FRCP(C)

This monograph is intended to be used as a portable reference for physiatrists and other professionals interested in the treatment of patients who have sustained a traumatic brain injury (TBI). Since brain injury is a dynamic process, the monograph is organized to help conceptualize rehabilitation care along a continuum from coma to community re-entry. Providing such care is expected to bring the physiatrist into collaborative treatment with other clinicians in several settings, ranging from acute inpatient medical-surgical units to outpatient rehabilitation centers and residential care facilities.

As the patient with a brain injury progresses in his hospitalization, the physiatrist is faced with coordinating the patient's rehabilitation treatment, not only with acute care clinicians, but also with a variety of rehabilitation professionals. The brain injured patient's rehabilitation treatment team may initially comprise only a physiatrist and perhaps a physical or occupational therapist. As the patient improves, however, other rehabilitation disciplines will become involved. Thus, at the time the brain injured patient is transferred to a rehabilitation unit he will likely be assigned a "core team," which may include a nurse, physical therapist, occupational therapist, speech-language pathologist, neuropsychologist, social worker, and case coordinator/discharge planner. The roles of the various rehabilitation professionals may change depending on the institution and capabilities of team members. For example, in some rehabilitation institutions, occupational therapists make recommendations regarding swallowing; in other institutions, this role is performed by speech pathologists.

The challenge to the physiatrist is to coordinate rehabilitation care. This requires communicating the patient's functional capabilities and requirements using terms and concepts that are understood by every member of the interdisciplinary team.

Two commonly used interdisciplinary scales to describe impairments associated with TBI include the Rancho Los Amigos Scale of Cognitive Functioning (Table 1) and the Glasgow Coma Scale (Table 2). The Rancho Scale was developed by rehabilitation professionals at Rancho Los Amigos Hospital in Downey, California. It proposes that most persons who have sustained moderate to severe brain injuries exhibit a relatively active process of recovery that can be predicted along a continuum of eight stages, or levels. Treatment strategies can be reasonably guided by the Rancho levels. While there are inherent flaws in any stage theory, there are advantages of using such a paradigm to conceptualize brain injury interventions.

The first three chapters of this monograph provide reviews of the epidemiology, pathophysiology and neurosurgical management of persons who have sustained a TBI. These initial chapters also serve as the background for the fourth chapter, which addresses the initial rehabilitation consultation.

As the patient's level of functioning improves, there will continue to be significant cognitive and behavioral impairments, and the importance of cognitive rehabilitation and behavioral management become paramount. The prominence of cognitive rehabilitation distinguishes brain injury rehabilitation from other specialized programs in rehabilitation. Cognition, for the purposes of this monograph, is operatively defined as the five domains of the mental process that are the focus of rehabilitation: attention, executive functions, language, memory and visual-spatial functions. Cognitive rehabilitation encompasses strategies that enhance spontaneous recovery or facilitate compensatory skills following a TBI.

Patients with TBI have both physical (e.g., transfers, mobility) and cognitive functional goals. Cognitive rehabilitation must be integrated with the physical rehabilitation program. For example, learning how to get dressed requires both manual dexterity and the ability to sequence tasks. Thus, chapters 5, 6 and 7 integrate cognitive rehabilitation with neuropsychological and neuropharmacological interventions in order to maximize treatment outcomes.

The next five chapters in the monograph are devoted to individual topics of special interest in brain injury rehabilitation: management of seizure disorders, spasticity, heterotopic ossification, contracture management, and community reintegration. The final two chapters discuss the assessment and treatment of mild traumatic brain injuries and pediatric brain injury rehabilitation, two other important areas of TBI.

The authors would like to emphasize that medicine is a constantly changing field. Although the indications, doses and side effects of the various medications discussed in this monograph were reviewed by the contributors, prescribing practitioners should consult an authoritative source prior to ordering any particular drug.

In many ways, the management of brain injury highlights the challenges rehabilitation clinicians encounter in their daily practice when treating a variety of diseases. Many of the terms used in TBI to categorize clinical phenomena do not have standard operationalized definitions. As well, there is a dearth of research demonstrating the superiority of one intervention vs. another. Thus, many of the management strategies outlined in this monograph reflect the current practices of the contributors in their respective institutions. Hopefully, by reading this monograph, clinicians will be inspired to organize and participate in studies that may elucidate a greater understanding of TBI.

Table 1
Rancho Los Amigos Scale of Cognitive Functioning

Level I	No Response	Patient appears to be in a deep sleep and is completely unresponsive to any stimuli presented to him.
Level II	Generalized Response	Patient reacts inconsistently and non-purposefully to stimuli in a nonspecific manner. Responses are limited in nature and are often the same regardless of stimuli presented. Responses may include physiological changes, gross body movements, and vocalization. Responses are likely to be delayed. The earliest response is to deep pain.
Level III	Localized Response	Patient reacts specifically but inconsistently to stimuli. Responses are directly related to the type of stimulus presented, as in turning the head toward a sound or focusing on an object presented. The patient may withdraw an extremity and vocalize when presented with a painful stimulus. He may follow simple commands in an inconsistent, delayed manner such as closing his eyes or squeezing or extending an extremity. Once external stimuli are removed, he may lie quietly. He may also show a vague awareness of self and body by responding to discomfort (e.g., pulling a nasogastric tube or catheter or resisting restraints). He may show a bias toward responding to some persons, especially family and friends, but not others.

Level IV	Confused-Agitated	Patient is in a heightened state of activity, with severely decreased ability to process information. He is detached from the present and responds primarily to his own internal confusion. Behavior is frequently bizarre and non-purposeful relative to his immediate environment. He may cry out or scream out of proportion to stimuli even after removal; may show aggressive behavior, attempt to remove restraints or tubes, or crawl out of bed in a purposeful manner. He does not discriminate among persons or objects and is unable to cooperate directly with treatment efforts. Verbalization is frequently incoherent or inappropriate to the environment. Confabulation may be present; he may be hostile. Gross attention to environment is brief and selective attention is often nonexistent. While aware of present events, patient lacks short-term recall and may be reacting to past events. He is unable to perform self-care activities without maximum assistance. If not disabled physically, he may perform automatic motor activities such as hitting, sitting, reaching and ambulating as part of his agitated state but not necessarily as a purposeful act or on request.
Level V	Confused-Inappropriate	Patient appears alert and is able to respond to simple commands fairly consistently. With increased complexity of commands or lack of any external structure, however, responses are non-purposeful, random or, at best, fragmented toward any desired goal. He may show agitated behavior, not on an internal basis as in Level IV, but rather as a result of external stimuli and usually out of proportion to the stimulus. The patient

		has gross attention to the environment, is highly distractible, and lacks ability to focus attention on a specific task without frequent redirection. With structure, he may be able to converse on a social-automatic level for short periods of time. Verbalization is often inappropriate; confabulation may be triggered by present events. Memory is severely impaired, with confusion of past and present in reaction to ongoing activity. Patient lacks initiation of functional tasks and often shows inappropriate use of objects without external direction. He may be able to perform previously learned tasks when structured for him but is unable to learn new information. He responds best to self, body, comfort and, often, family members. The patient can perform self-care activities with assistance and may accomplish feeding with supervision. Management on the unit is often a problem if the patient is physically mobile, as he may wander off either randomly or with the vague intention of "going home."
Level VI	Confused-Appropriate	Patient shows goal-directed behavior, but is dependent on external input for direction. Response to discomfort is appropriate, and he is able to tolerate unpleasant stimuli (e.g., a nasogastric tube, when need is explained). He follows simple directions consistently and shows carry-over (recall) for tasks he has relearned (e.g., self care). He is at least supervised with old learning; new learning requires maximal training; there is little carry-over. Responses may be incorrect due to memory problems, but are appropriate to the situation due to preservation of "automatic" responses.

		Patients at this level may show decreased ability to process information, with little or no anticipation or prediction of events. Past memories show more depth and detail than recent memory. The patient may show beginning awareness of this situation by realizing he doesn't know an answer. He no longer wanders and is consistently oriented to time and place. Selective attention to tasks may be impaired, especially with difficult tasks and in unstructured settings, but is now functional for common daily activities. He may show vague recognition of some staff and has increased awareness of self, family and basic needs.
Level VII	Automatic-Appropriate	Patient appears and behaves appropriately while being oriented within hospital settings. Goes through daily routine automatically but robot-like, with minimal to absent confusion and has shallow recall of what he has been doing. He shows increased awareness of self, body, family, food, people and interaction with the environment. He has superficial awareness of but lacks insight into his condition. He has decreased judgment and problem solving abilities and lacks realistic planning for his future. He shows carry-over for new learning at a decreased rate. He requires at least minimal supervision for learning and safety measures. He is independent in self-care activities and supervised in home and community skills for safety. With structure, he is able to initiate tasks or social and recreational activities in which he now has interest. His judgment remains impaired. Prevocational evaluation and counseling may be indicated.

Level VIII	Purposeful- Appropriate	Patient is alert and oriented, is able to recall and integrate past and recent events, and is aware of and responsive to societal norms. He shows carry-over for new learning if acceptable to him and his life role and needs no supervision once activities are learned. Within his physical capabilities, he is independent in home and community skills. Vocational rehabilitation, to determine ability to return as a contributor to society, perhaps in a new capacity, is indicated. He may continue to show decreases relative to premorbid abilities in quality and rate of processing, abstract reasoning, tolerance for stress, and judgment in emergencies or unusual circumstances. His social, emotional and intellectual capacities may continue to be at a decreased level for him, but functional within society.

Source: Nalkmus D, Booth BJ, Kodimer C. Rehabilitation of the head injured adult: comprehensive cognitive management. Downey, CA: Professional Staff Association of Rancho Los Amigos Hospital, Inc.; 1980.

Table 2
Glasgow Coma Scale

Patient's Response	Score
Eye opening	
Eyes open spontaneously	4
Eyes open when spoken to	3
Eyes open to painful stimulation	2
Eyes do not open	1
Motor	
Follows commands	6
Makes localizing movements to pain	5
Makes withdrawal movements to pain	4
Flexor (decorticate) posturing to pain	3
Extensor (decerebrate) posturing to pain	2
No motor response to pain	1
Verbal	
Oriented to place and date	5
Converses but is disoriented	4
Utters inappropriate words, not conversing	3
Makes incomprehensible nonverbal sounds	2
Not vocalizing	1
Total: _____	

Table 3
Severity of Traumatic Brain Injury

	Glasgow Coma Scale Score
Severe TBI	less than 9
Moderate TBI	9 to 12
Mild TBI	greater than 12

Chapter 1

Epidemiology of Traumatic Brain Injury

Buck H. Woo, PhD
Georgia Thoidis, MA, MPH

Traumatic brain injury (TBI) represents a significant social and financial burden on the affected individuals, their families, and the broader community. It is difficult, however, to accurately describe the epidemiology of TBI for two reasons. First, there is an inconsistency in the definition and classification of TBI in the various studies and data bases. Several terms are used to describe TBI, and the various terms may indicate very different types of injuries. Second, many of the epidemiological studies are based on data collected from hospital charts, physician progress notes, death certificates, or insurance billing records. Yet, many people who suffer from mild TBI are not evaluated by a physician or assessed in a hospital emergency department. Therefore, these individuals are frequently not included in the epidemiological studies. In addition, many victims of trauma die at the scene of injury or during transport to the hospital. The cause of death of many of these patients is not always clearly defined on the death certificate, and many of these individuals did suffer from an unrecognized TBI. These fatal TBI are not accounted for in epidemiological studies. Given these limitations, estimates of incidence and prevalence of TBI are inconsistent and variable among studies.

Incidence and Prevalence

Several studies have attempted to determine the incidence of TBI in the United States. The National Health Interview Survey estimates that 1.5 to 2 million people suffer TBI each year in the U.S., approximately one million of whom are treated in hospital emergency departments. Of these, 230,000 are hospitalized and 51,000 die. A recent report describing data collected from four state health departments (Colorado, Missouri, Oklahoma and Utah), which used guidelines developed by the U.S. Centers for Disease Control and Prevention (CDC) for TBI surveillance, determined that the annual combined TBI incidence for these states was 102 cases per 100,000 people. These agencies used hospital discharge and mortality data to identify all cases of TBI.

Although data are limited, it is useful to separately address mild, moderate and severe TBI. Severe TBI is defined by a Glasgow Coma Scale (GCS) score of less than 9 obtained within 48 hours of injury. Using this GCS threshold, the incidence of severe TBI is 14 for every 100,000 people, with a case fatality rate of 58 percent. The incidence of moderate TBI (a GCS score between 9 and 12) is 15 per 100,000, while mild TBI (a GCS score greater than 12) is 131 per 100,000.

A recent long-term study, conducted by the CDC, estimated that the annual incidence of hospitalization associated with TBI was 98 per 100,000 people in 1995 (down 51% from 199 per 100,000 in 1980). In a different study, Thurman and Guerrero evaluated the rate of hospitalization for severe, moderate and mild TBI. The rate of hospitalization for severe TBI was 19 per 100,000 (up 90% from 10 per 100,000 in 1980), 21 per 100,000 for moderate TBI (down 19% from 26 per 100,000), and 51 per 100,000 for mild TBI (down 61% from 131 per 100,000). The study estimated the annual rate of TBI-related visits to hospital emergency departments at 395 per 100,000 people.

Most estimates of prevalence are based on data derived from hospital records. The National Institutes of Health Consensus Development Panel on Rehabilitation of Persons with TBI estimated that there are between 2.5 and 6.5 million Americans living with TBI-related disabilities.

Risk Factors

Certain segments of the population are at higher risk of sustaining a TBI than others. In general, younger, poor, unmarried, minority, inner-city men are the most likely to suffer traumatic brain injuries. Other risk factors include history of substance abuse and previous TBI.

Gender

For persons of all ages, males are more than twice as likely as females to have a TBI. Using data from the National Hospital Discharge Survey, the CDC determined that males, in 1995, suffered TBI at a rate of 130 per 100,000 (down from 260 per 100,000 in 1981) and that women suffered from TBI at a rate of 71 per 100,000 (down from 145 per 100,000). For the years 1979 through 1992, the National Center for Health Statistics determined the male-to-female ratio for TBI to be 3.4-to-1.

Age

The risk of TBI is greatest among those 15 to 24 years of age (250 per 100,000). Mortality rates from TBI are highest in this group as well (33 per 100,000). The incidence of TBI also peaks in the elderly, especially those over 65 years of age. TBI-associated death rate for those over 65 is 31 per 100,000. The male-to-female ratio decreases in the elderly.

Mechanisms of Injury

The leading cause of TBI is motor vehicle collisions, which account for about 50 percent of all traumatic brain injuries. The CDC reports that motor vehicle-related TBI occur in 114 of every 100,000 people between the ages of 15 and 24.

Falls are the second leading cause of TBI and account for about 21 percent of all cases, with the highest rates attributed to the very young and the elderly. Falls are the leading cause of TBI in the population 75 and older (120 per 100,000).

Firearms are the third leading cause of TBI, accounting for about 12 percent of all brain injuries. The incidence of gunshot-related fatal TBI is six times higher among men than it is among women. Firearms are one of the leading causes of TBI among those 25 to 34 years of age.

Sports and recreational activities contribute to 10 percent of all brain injuries. TBI related to sports are most common between the ages of 5 and 64, with the highest incidence occurring between 5 and 24 years of age. Football, basketball, baseball and wrestling account for the greatest number of sports-related TBI.

The remaining TBI are classified in the "other" category, including work-related accidents and injuries of unknown origin.

Cost

It is difficult to accurately determine the associated costs of traumatic brain injuries. An estimate of cost should include the direct and indirect medical expenditures, as well as loss of current and future earnings. In addition, a complete estimate should assign a value for the expenditure of energies of paid and unpaid caregivers. Furthermore, it is difficult to compensate for the affected individuals' pain and suffering, as well as the additional psychosocial burdens placed on family members. Very few analyses have been done on the loss of potential income, the cost of acute care, and the continued expenses of rehabilitation and medical care. Max, MacKenzie and Rice divided the cost of TBI into three categories: direct cost (expenditures for hospital and nursing home care, physician services, drugs, and other goods and services), morbidity cost (injury-related work loss and disability), and mortality cost (losses resulting from premature death). In 1985 dollars, the annual direct costs of TBI were estimated at $4.5 billion; morbidity costs were estimated at $20.6 billion; and mortality costs were estimated at $12.7 billion. The mortality costs represent a loss of 1.4 million life years, or 38 years per death.

Trends

There are several ongoing trends in the epidemiology of traumatic brain injury that are worthy of note. First, the incidence of TBI appears to be declining. Second, while the focus of TBI prevention appears to be in other areas, the incidence of death due to firearms-related TBI is rising.

Preventive efforts, such as the use of airbags and seat belts in motor vehicles, enforcement of drunk driving laws, and the use of helmets in sports and recreational activities, have reduced the incidence of head injuries, but the magnitude is difficult to determine. A National Hospital Discharge Survey indicated that the number of discharges of patients diagnosed with acute head injury decreased from 309,000 in 1979 to 160,000 in 1993. The greatest decline was for those patients diagnosed with concussions. The overall mortality rate from head injuries fell 22 percent from 1979 to 1992, and the mortality due to motor vehicle crashes dropped 42 percent.

Finally, there is evidence that lengths of stay in acute hospitals and inpatient rehabilitation facilities are generally declining. A survey conducted by the Traumatic Brain Injury Model Systems suggests that lengths of stay in acute hospitals have declined by 50 percent, from 30 days in 1989 to 15 days in 1996. In addition, the average length of stay in inpatient rehabilitation facilities has decreased by 38 percent, from 52 days to 32 days during the same period. The reduction in inpatient days places increasing demands on resources in the community to care for persons who may otherwise still be hospitalized.

Suggested Readings:

NIH Consensus Development Panel on Rehabilitation of Persons with Traumatic Brain Injury. Journal of the American Medical Association 1999; 282(10):974-983.

Centers for Disease Control and Prevention. Traumatic brain injury — Colorado, Missouri, Oklahoma, and Utah, 1990 - 1993. Morbidity and Mortality Weekly Review 1997; 46(1):8-11.

Torner JC, Choi S, Barnes TY. Epidemiology of head injuries. In: Marion DW, editor. Traumatic brain injury. New York: Thieme Medical Publishers; 1998; 9-25.

Kraus JF, Black MA, Hessol N, Ley P, Rokaw W, Sullivan C, Bowers S, Knowlton S, Marshall L. The incidence of acute brain injury and serious impairment in a defined population. American Journal of Epidemiology 1984 Feb; 119(2):186-201.

Thurman D, Guerrero J. Trends in hospital associated with traumatic brain injury. Journal of the American Medical Association 1999; 282(10):954-957.

Sosin DM, Sniezek JE, Waxweiler RJ. Trends in death associated with traumatic brain injury, 1979 through 1992: success and failure. Journal of the American Medical Association 1995; 273(22):1778-1780.

Powell JW, Barber-Foss KD. Traumatic brain injury in high school athletes. Journal of the American Medical Association 1999; 282(10):958-963.

Max W, MacKenzie EJ, Rice DP. Head injuries: costs and consequences. Journal of Head Trauma Rehabilitation 1991; 6(2):76-91.

The Traumatic Brain Injury Model Systems National Data Center. www.tbims.org.

Chapter 2

Pathophysiology of Traumatic Brain Injury

David Burke, MD, MA
Joe I. Ordia, MD, FACS

Traumatic brain injuries (TBI) are insults to the brain by an external physical force, which cause either temporary or permanent impairments, partial or total functional disability, or psychosocial maladjustment. TBI can be divided into primary injuries, which occur immediately at the time of the trauma, and secondary injuries, which begin immediately after the trauma and continue for an indefinite period of time. The clinical manifestations of TBI can range from a concussion to profound coma and even death.

Primary Injury

Primary injuries occur immediately at the time of impact and are associated with acceleration-deceleration and rotational forces. Primary injuries can be focal or diffuse. Focal injuries include skull fractures, intracranial hematomas, cortical contusions, lacerations, and penetrating wounds. Alternatively, a primary brain injury can be diffuse in nature, with widespread axonal involvement (i.e., diffuse axonal injury).

Skull Fractures

Skull fractures can be divided into fractures of the vault or base. Skull fractures are associated with an increased risk of brain injury, hematoma, and cranial nerve damage. Neurosurgical considerations with respect to skull fractures are discussed in chapter 3.

Cranial vault fractures can be described as closed or compound, linear or stellate, non-depressed or depressed. Closed fractures do not have any communication to the outside environment. In contrast, compound fractures communicate with the outside environment (e.g., fracture beneath a scalp laceration or fracture in continuity with an air sinus). Linear fractures imply a break in a single line that usually occurs over the lateral convexity of the skull, whereas stellate injuries have star-like fracture lines. Depressed skull fractures occur when the fragments are displaced inward.

Basal skull fractures (Figure 2.1) often coincide with trauma over a large surface area. Impact over a thick region of the skull may produce very little change in the immediate area, but as the energy of the impact dissipates to the thinner regions of the skull base a corresponding fracture may result.

Basal skull fractures frequently occur in the cribriform plate of the ethmoid bone. This may result in rhinorrhea (see chapter 11). TBI can also result from a fracture of the petrous portion of the temporal bone, which may result in post-auricular ecchymosis and hemotympanum. Longitudinal temporal bone fractures are more likely to result in contusion or laceration of the seventh cranial nerve (CN), whereas transverse fractures are more likely to injure the eighth cranial nerve. CN VII palsy may lead to facial paralysis and disorder of taste. CN VIII compromise may result in diminished hearing, dizziness and vertigo.

Auditory and Vestibular Dysfunction

Blows to the temporal region may result in hearing loss that may not always be associated with a basal skull fracture. Both conductive and sensorineural hearing loss are possible. Causes of conductive hearing loss include tympanic perforation, hemotympanum, and ossicular disruption. Common causes of sensorineural hearing loss include acute cochlear concussion and perilymphatic fistula.

Another condition associated with TBI is benign paroxysmal positional vertigo, or BPPV. In this condition, calcium carbonate crystals become dislodged from the macula of the utricle and enter the posterior semicircular canal. This results in episodic vertigo that is provoked by rapid head movements. The Dix-Hallpike maneuver is a useful diagnostic test. Patients may respond to an Epley repositioning maneuver.

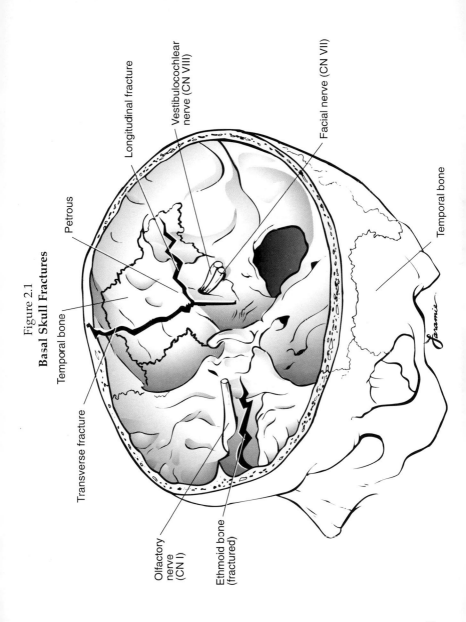

Figure 2.1
Basal Skull Fractures

Longitudinal fracture

Vestibulocochlear nerve (CN VIII)

Facial nerve (CN VII)

Petrous

Temporal bone

Temporal bone

Temporal bone

Transverse fracture

Olfactory nerve (CN I)

Ethmoid bone (fractured)

21

Intracranial Hemorrhages

Intracranial hemorrhages (epidural, subdural, intracerebral and subarachnoid) are a major concern with respect to TBI. Hematomas can cause further damage to the brain by placing direct pressure on underlying brain structures (Figure 2.2) or they may cause a portion of the brain to herniate and compress the brain stem (Figure 2.3).

Epidural hematomas (EDH) are caused by an impact to the head, which results in laceration of the dural veins and arteries. Alternatively, the source of blood can be from diploic veins in the marrow of the skull. EDH are usually associated with a tear in the middle meningeal artery and often, but not always, occur in the presence of a skull fracture. The underlying brain injury is usually not severe if treated promptly; however, if an EDH is related to an arterial laceration, it is able to evolve quickly and can result in rapid deterioration and death.

Subdural hematomas (SDH) occur from injuries to a cortical bridging vein or pial artery. SDH are common in severe brain injuries. The prognosis is poor, and the mortality is high (60 to 80%) because of the severity of the underlying parenchymal injury.

Intracerebral hemorrhages occur within the brain parenchyma. They arise from lacerations of the brain or coalescence of contusional hemorrhages. They occur mostly in the frontal and temporal lobes, but may be found in the cerebellum and brain stem.

Subarachnoid hemorrhages (SAH) occur frequently with TBI and may be related to underlying hemorrhagic contusions. The pathology of traumatic SAH is different from SAH related to ruptured aneurysms. Specifically, SAH are the result of shearing of the microvessels in the subarachnoid space. These injuries, if not associated with other structural pathology, have a relatively benign course. On occasion, a traumatic SAH can lead to communicating hydrocephalus as blood products can cause obstruction of the arachnoid villi. Rarely, a clot in the third or fourth ventricle can lead to non-communicating hydrocephalus, which is discussed later in this chapter. Neurosurgical considerations with respect to intracranial hematomas are discussed in chapter 3.

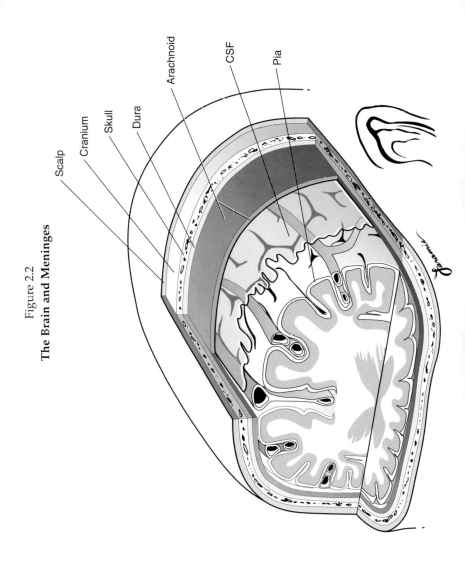

Figure 2.2
The Brain and Meninges

Scalp

Cranium

Skull

Dura

Arachnoid

CSF

Pia

Figure 2.3
Intracranial Hemorrhages

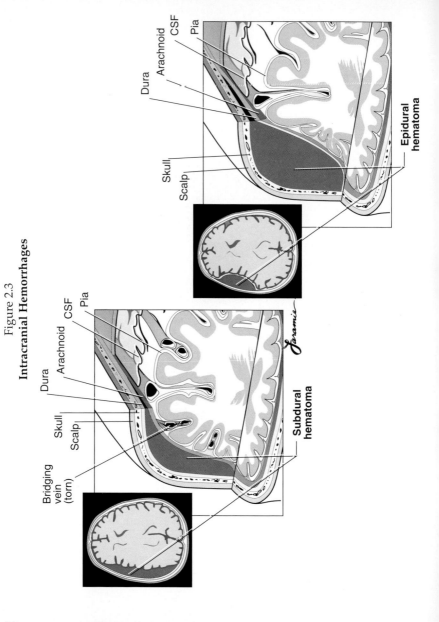

CSF
Pia
Arachnoid
Dura
Skull
Scalp
Epidural hematoma

CSF
Pia
Arachnoid
Dura
Skull
Scalp
Bridging vein (torn)
Subdural hematoma

Cortical Contusions

Cortical contusions are considered a specific characteristic of TBI. In some cases, cortical contusions are very involved and may extend through the cortex and into the subcortical white matter. The distribution of cortical contusions is somewhat predictable due to the bony protrusions that the brain strikes along the interior wall of the skull. The movement of the brain in the skull, caused by acceleration-deceleration and rotational forces, causes certain cortical areas to be more susceptible to injury. For example, coup and contrecoup injuries occur when the head is in motion and strikes a stationary object or surface. The coup injury occurs as the brain pushes forward in the direction of the impact striking the skull. The contrecoup injury, which is frequently more severe, occurs as the brain rebounds in a contralateral direction from the original direction of the impact. These contusions usually occur bilaterally and are distributed in frontopolar, orbitalfrontal, anterior temporal, and lateral temporal regions (Figure 2.4).

Damage to these areas manifests as cognitive and behavioral changes, which can significantly impact the patient's rehabilitation. These brain-behavior relationships are discussed in greater detail with respect to neuropsychology interventions in chapter 6. Clinically, cortical contusions may produce focal neurological deficits and seizures.

Diffuse Axonal Injury

Diffuse axonal injury (DAI) refers to extensive damage to the white matter of the brain. DAI occurs as nerve cells are torn from each other as the brain bounces and twists in the skull at the time of injury (Figure 2.5). There is shearing of the white matter with widespread mechanical disruption of axons and myelin sheaths in the cerebral hemispheres, corpus callosum, brain stem, and cerebellar peduncles. Usually, there is a deep and prolonged coma from the moment of impact. It may be difficult to always appreciate DAI from CT and MRI studies. On occasion, these investigations may demonstrate petechial hemorrhages. In contrast to cortical contusions, which are associated with falls and direct blows to the head, DAI is consistent with high-speed acceleration-deceleration injuries, such as those caused by motor vehicle collisions.

Penetrating Brain Injuries

Penetrating brain injuries are produced by gunshot wounds and other missiles and non-missiles (e.g., assault with a nailed board). High-velocity (>2,000 feet/second) missiles inflict the most damage. The shock waves produced upon skull penetration produce a cylinder of damaged brain tissue up to 30 times the diameter of the bullet. These shock waves may be transmitted to the brain stem and can result in rapid death. The kinetic energy determines the injury potential, and it increases exponentially with velocity

Figure 2.4
Areas of Cortical Contusion

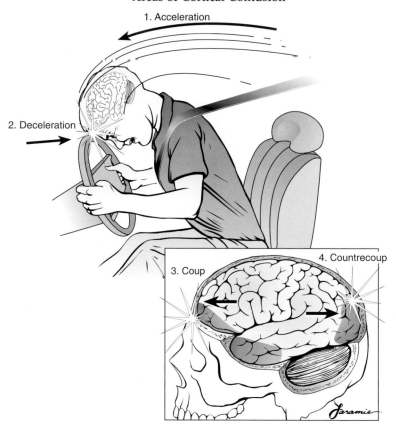

1. Acceleration

2. Deceleration

3. Coup

4. Countrecoup

(i.e., energy transmitted = one-half mass of missile x square of velocity). In addition, bullets often fragment, causing damage in multiple directions, and skin and hair are driven into the brain, acting as a source for infection.

Secondary Injury

Secondary injuries are the biochemical and physiological sequelae of the primary brain insult that evolve over a period of hours or days. They cause cerebral ischemia and tissue hypoxia. The effects of intracranial hematomas and increased intracranial pressure (ICP) on the secondary injury are discussed in chapter 3. The biochemical changes are discussed here.

Figure 2.5
Diffuse Axonal Injury

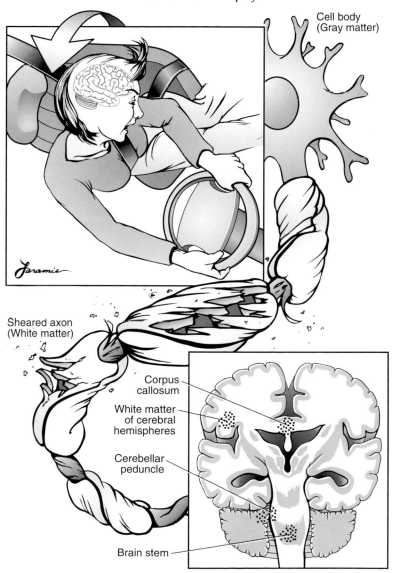

Cell body
(Gray matter)

Sheared axon
(White matter)

Corpus
callosum

White matter
of cerebral
hemispheres

Cerebellar
peduncle

Brain stem

Neurochemical and Cellular Events

Neurochemical and cellular events, which cause further damage following TBI, are characterized by complex biochemical processes that are usually triggered by the failure of physiologic autoregulatory mechanisms. Focal ischemia, which occurs in approximately 90 percent of TBI cases, is implicated in initiating many of the toxic neurochemical processes. Increased levels of excitatory amino acids, endogenous opioid peptides, and acetylcholine are among the neurochemical agents that contribute to secondary brain damage (Table 1).

Table 1
Mechanisms of Secondary Brain Injury Following TBI

Biochemical Process	Toxicity
Focal ischemia	Lactic acidosis, excitatory amino acids, extracellular potassium
Excitatory amino acids	Oxygen free radicals
Cytokines	Inflammation
Acetylcholine	Increased sensitivity to ischemia
Endogenous opioid peptides	Decreased cerebral perfusion
Catecholamines	Ischemia
Oxygen free radicals	Edema, hyperemia
Lipid peroxides	Edema, hyperemia
Extracellular potassium	Edema
Increased calcium entry into cells	Oxygen free radicals
Decreased intracellular magnesium	Increased calcium entry into cells

Intracranial Pressure Effects

Elevations of ICP as a secondary effect of brain injury are associated with poorer functional outcomes, especially if pressure is beyond 40 mm Hg. Better outcomes are noted if increased ICP is not accompanied by a midline shift. Increased ICP contributes to cerebral ischemia and hypoxia, and may be associated with cerebral edema, hydrocephalus, and herniation syndromes. Neurosurgical management of these conditions is addressed in chapter 3.

Cerebral Edema

Cerebral edema or swelling can be focal or diffuse. Localized edema can occur at the focal areas of the brain contusion or it can be diffuse, with generalized swelling of the entire brain. Brain swelling is attributed to disruption of the blood-brain barrier and impairment of vasomotor autoregulation with concomitant dilation of cerebral blood vessels. Consequently, water and electrolytes enter the adjacent white matter.

Hydrocephalus

The flow of cerebrospinal fluid (CSF) begins with its secretion from the choroid plexus of the lateral ventricles in the brain. The production of CSF is largely continuous (500 ml/day) in the lateral ventricles, where it then passes through the interventricular foramina and combines with CSF produced in the third ventricle. It then passes through the cerebral aqueduct into the fourth ventricle. Additional fluid is added here from the choroid plexus of the fourth ventricle and escapes by way of one median and two lateral foramina located in the roof of the fourth ventricle into the subarachnoid space surrounding the lower brain stem. CSF in the cranial subarachnoid space is continuous with spinal CSF. Cerebrospinal fluid is absorbed largely through the arachnoid villi projecting into the superior sagittal sinus. Some absorption also takes place at small villi close to the exit of spinal nerves from the spinal dura (Figure 2.6).

Hydrocephalus ("water on the brain") is the dilation of the cerebral ventricular system. It occurs when the normal flow of CSF is impaired, leading to an abnormal accumulation of fluid. Less often, it is due to excessive production of CSF. Hydrocephalus is known to compromise cerebral perfusion, particularly in the frontal and periventricular regions. It can be divided into communicating and non-communicating hydrocephalus.

Figure 2.6
Flow of Cerebrospinal Fluid

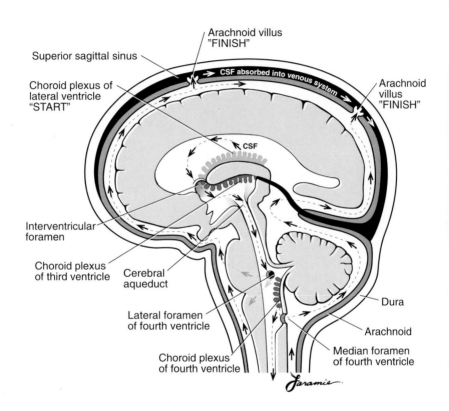

Arachnoid villus "FINISH"

Superior sagittal sinus

Choroid plexus of lateral ventricle "START"

CSF absorbed into venous system

Arachnoid villus "FINISH"

CSF

Interventricular foramen

Choroid plexus of third ventricle

Cerebral aqueduct

Lateral foramen of fourth ventricle

Choroid plexus of fourth ventricle

Dura

Arachnoid

Median foramen of fourth ventricle

Communicating hydrocephalus is the most frequently occurring type in TBI. Ventricular enlargement usually involves all components of the ventricular system. The presence of blood products causes impairment of the circulation of CSF through the subarachnoid space and its absorption into the blood stream through the arachnoid villi.

Non-communicating hydrocephalus occurs when the CSF obstruction takes place within the ventricular system. For example, a blood clot in the interventricular foramen, third ventricle, cerebral aqueduct, or fourth ventricle can result in non-communicating hydrocephalus. In TBI, non-communicating hydrocephalus occurs much less frequently than communicating hydrocephalus.

Brain Herniation Syndromes

Brain herniation syndromes are pathological changes that can damage the brain stem by direct mechanical compression or intracranial hypertension. The mortality for brain stem herniation is high. Brain herniation syndromes occur in three distinguishable patterns: subfalcine, transtentorial and cerebellar (Figure 2.7).

Subfalcine herniation occurs when the cingulate gyrus of the frontal lobe is pushed under and across the falx to the side opposite the mass lesion. As herniation progresses, the patient is agitated and can rapidly become comatose.

Transtentorial herniation refers to compression of the midbrain by an expanding mass that displaces the uncus and hippocampal gyrus of the temporal lobe into the tentorial notch. The ipsilateral third cranial nerve and cerebral peduncle are compressed, resulting in ipsilateral dilated and fixed pupil and contralateral hemiparesis.

A mass or hematoma in the posterior fossa can cause the tonsil of the cerebellum to herniate into the foramen magnum and compress the medulla. Bradycardia and respiratory arrest occur rapidly.

Conclusion

The pathophysiology of TBI is reflected by complex interactive changes at both the neuroanatomical and cellular levels. It is best conceptualized as a dynamic process that is only partially understood, but can be influenced in many instances by medical intervention and rehabilitation treatments.

Figure 2.7
Brain Herniation Syndromes

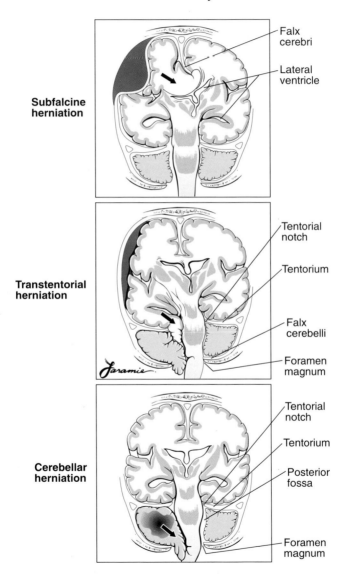

Subfalcine herniation

Falx cerebri

Lateral ventricle

Transtentorial herniation

Tentorial notch

Tentorium

Falx cerebelli

Foramen magnum

Jaramie

Cerebellar herniation

Tentorial notch

Tentorium

Posterior fossa

Foramen magnum

Suggested Readings:

Auerbach S. The pathophysiology of traumatic brain injury. In: Horn J, Cope N. Traumatic brain injury, physical medicine and rehabilitation: state of the art reviews (vol. 3, no. 1). Philadelphia: Hanley & Belfus, Inc.; 1989.

Horn L, Zasler N. Medical rehabilitation of traumatic brain injury. Philadelphia: Hanley & Belfus, Inc.; 1996.

Geisler F, Saloman M. The head injury patient. In: Siegal JH, editor. Trauma emergency surgery and critical care. New York: Churchill Livingstone; 1987; 919-46.

Chapter 3

Surgical Management of Traumatic Brain Injury

Joe I. Ordia, MD, FACS

To achieve successful clinical outcomes, patients with traumatic brain injuries (TBI) require a comprehensive system of care that begins with a well-organized emergency medical service. Injured patients require a trauma team that includes a variety of specialists, including neurosurgeons, general surgeons, emergency physicians, and orthopedists. In addition, a properly staffed institution with skilled and experienced nurses and therapists is essential. Access to radiological and laboratory investigations on a 24-hour basis is also necessary.

Acute TBI is a dynamic condition, and patients can rapidly deteriorate. As such, a comprehensive initial examination and meaningful serial evaluation are essential for the early recognition and prompt management of treatable pathology. A comprehensive assessment includes a thorough history, physical examination, and review of pertinent radiological and laboratory investigations. Cardinal elements of the history can be obtained from the patient and/or witnesses at the scene of injury (i.e., family, emergency medical service personnel, etc.).

The level of consciousness is the single most important indicator of the severity of brain injury. Therefore, it is important to ascertain, if possible, the initial and subsequent levels of consciousness and to document the findings. The mechanism of injury should also be determined (i.e., fall, motor vehicle collision, assault, etc.). Physical examination at the time of acute presentation may be limited by patient cooperation and the presence of comorbidity. Essential elements during the initial examination include level of consciousness, which may be summarized by the Glasgow Coma Scale (GCS), pupillary size and response, and blood pressure and heart rate. The ability to speak, follow commands, and move the extremities is noted. Decerebrate and decorticate posturing should be noted if present. A more thorough physical examination that evaluates mental status, cranial nerves, reflexes, muscle strength and sensation, however, may be performed at a later time. CT scan of the head is the radiological test of choice in the evaluation of acute TBI. On occasion, X-rays of the skull, MRI, and cerebral angiography may be indicated. For patients with severe TBI, laboratory studies should include blood gases, hematocrit, electrolytes, alcohol level, and a toxic screen. Alcohol is a factor in one-half of motor vehicle collisions and in many cases of assault.

Severe TBI is rarely an isolated event. More than 50 percent of TBI have associated traumatic injuries, such as spinal fracture, long bone fracture, lacerated abdominal organ, and perforated abdominal viscus, that must be identified and treated. The first objective of the trauma team is to address the "ABCs" of trauma care (i.e., airway, breathing, circulation with spine precautions). The neurosurgeon's foremost objective is to treat the primary brain injury and to minimize and treat the secondary injury. Primary injury occurs at the moment of impact and includes focal conditions such as cerebral contusions, brain lacerations, and skull fractures. Patients may present with focal neurological deficits and seizures. Emergency surgical treatment may be required to evacuate large contusional brain hemorrhages, for placement of an intracranial pressure (ICP) monitoring device, or to elevate a depressed skull fracture. Secondary injury arises for the most part from cerebral ischemia and neuronal hypoxemia. Elevated ICP and intracranial hematomas are the most common causes of secondary injury. Prompt administration of osmotic diuretics and evacuation of hematoma can prevent secondary injury and reduce morbidity and mortality.

Indications for Admission to Hospital for Observation

- altered level of consciousness
- prolonged loss of consciousness
- continuous nausea and vomiting
- post-traumatic seizures
- severe headaches
- focal neurological signs
- skull fracture less than 24 hours old
- penetrating brain injury
- cerebrospinal fluid (CSF) rhinorrhea or otorrhea
- cerebral contusion, swelling or intracranial hematoma.

Skull Fracture

Anatomically, skull fractures can be divided into fractures of the vault or base (see chapter 2). Fractures of the cranial vault can generally be detected on plain X-rays or on CT scans. The likelihood of a brain injury, intracranial hematoma, and cranial nerve (CN) injury is increased in the presence of a skull fracture.

Fractures of the cranial vault are recognized as being closed or compound, linear or stellate, non-depressed or depressed. Linear fractures usually heal without neurosurgical intervention. With depressed skull fractures, one or more fracture fragments may be hinged inward, and bone fragments may lacerate the dura and penetrate the brain, causing contusion or hemorrhage. The brain may become contaminated, leading to meningitis or brain abscess. Basal skull fractures are associated with signs of CSF rhinorrhea or otorrhea, hemotympanum, retroauricular ecchymosis (Battle sign), and periorbital ecchymosis (raccoon sign). Basal skull fractures may be associated with cranial nerve abnormalities (e.g., diminished sense of smell due to CN I injury or facial palsy due to CN VII injury).

In general, compound fractures require exploration. Fractures depressed greater than the thickness of the skull require debridement and elevation. Persistent CSF rhinorrhea or otorrhea demand surgical repair of the dural fistula. Accessible retained bone fragments should be removed. If a fracture involves a venous sinus, surgical intervention may be unwise because of the risk of bleeding.

Surgical Management of Intracranial Hemorrhages

Neurosurgical treatment of intracranial hemorrhages is a fundamental component of acute TBI treatment. A review of the pathophysiology of intracranial hematomas is provided in chapter 2. This chapter will focus on neurosurgical treatment and management.

Epidural hematomas (EDH) are found in 1 percent of TBI admissions and in 10 percent of severe TBI. The clinical presentation is variable. In the "classic" case, there is a brief loss of consciousness at the time of injury, followed by a lucid interval during which the patient appears alert after recovering from the initial concussion, and then lapses into a coma as the hematoma expands. Some patients will experience persistent coma from the time of injury, but there are also situations in which there is no loss of consciousness. CT imaging shows the location and size of the EDH and the degree of brain compression. EDH are usually located in the temporal region, where they are frequently associated with laceration of the middle meningeal artery by a skull fracture. EDH following a skull fracture can occur from diploic bleeding. Craniotomy permits evacuation of the hematoma and control of hemostasis.

Subdural hematomas (SDH) represent a collection of blood between the dura and the brain. Acute SDH are present in 30 percent of severe TBI. The untoward effects of an acute subdural hematoma are related to the associated cerebral injury and the mass effect, which often leads to herniation (see chapter 2) or a reduction of cerebral perfusion. The blood also has a direct toxic effect on underlying brain tissue. SDH are associated with parenchymal lesions such as lacerations and contusions. The clinical signs and symptoms of SDH include alteration of consciousness, pupillary abnormalities, and abnormal motor response (decerebrate and decorticate posturing, hemiparesis or hemiplegia).

A large intracranial hemorrhage can lead to elevated ICP and brain herniation (transtentorial, subfalcine or cerebellar). Thus, most large hemorrhages should be evacuated. At the time of surgery, necrotic and severely contused brain tissue may be removed. This must be done with caution, however, as removal of tissue in "elegant" areas may result in further neurological deficit.

Placement of an ICP monitoring device, also called an "ICP bolt" (Figure 3.1), after evacuation of the hematoma is a helpful adjunct for postoperative management. If the SDH is small and not producing significant mass effect, surgery may not be necessary.

By themselves, *subarachnoid hemorrhages* (SAH) due to TBI have a relatively benign course. There are occasions when traumatic SAH become the source of communicating hydrocephalus, as blood products may cause obstruction of the arachnoid villi (see chapter 2). In addition, in some rare instances a clot in the aqueduct or the third or fourth ventricle can cause acute non-communicating hydrocephalus, which may initially require treatment with a ventriculostomy (Figure 3.2) and, later on, a ventriculoperitoneal shunt.

Penetrating Brain Injury

Penetrating brain injuries may be caused by missiles (e.g., gunshot wounds) or non-missiles (e.g., assault with a hammer). High-velocity (>2,000 feet/second) missiles inflict the most damage. The shock waves produced upon skull penetration are transmitted to the brain stem and can result in rapid death. The goals of surgical treatment include removal of foreign bodies (e.g., bullets, skull fragments, hair, etc.), as well as repairing the dura.

Management of Elevated Intracranial Pressure

One of the most important goals of neurosurgical management is to maintain normal intracranial pressure. As explained in chapter 2, elevated ICP is associated with poorer functional outcomes, contributes to cerebral ischemia, and is associated with cerebral edema and herniation syndromes.

A monitoring device (Figure 3.1) can facilitate the continuous monitoring of ICP. This device can be placed in the subdural space, brain parenchyma, or ventricle. It is also possible to place a pressure-recording device in the extradural space; however, these are not as accurate as those in the ventricle.

The decision to place an ICP monitoring device should be individualized. ICP monitoring in patients with a GCS score of 8 or less after resuscitation and an abnormal head CT is a widely accepted practice. It may not be necessary, however, if the CT scan is normal or shows minimal mass effect. The neurosurgeon may also elect not to monitor ICP if the patient has a GCS score of 3 and minimal brain stem function. The therapeutic goal is to keep ICP at 15 mm Hg or below and maintain cerebral perfusion and oxygenation.

Figure 3.1
ICP Montoring Device

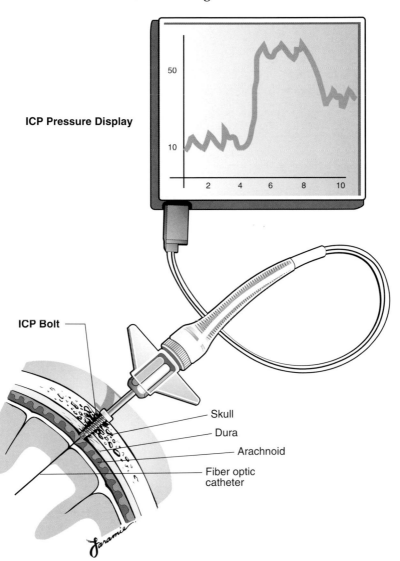

ICP Pressure Display

ICP Bolt

Skull

Dura

Arachnoid

Fiber optic
catheter

Figure 3.2
Ventriculostomy

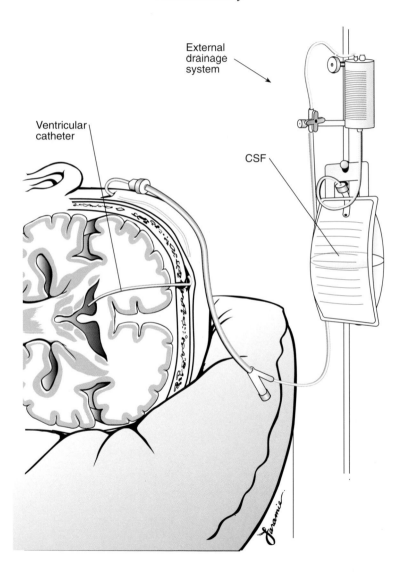

External
drainage
system

Ventricular
catheter

CSF

Elevated ICP in acute TBI is usually due to focal intracranial hematoma or cerebral vasocongestion and diffuse cerebral edema from loss of autoregulation and breakdown of the blood-brain barrier. On occasion, hydrocephalus can cause elevated ICP. Therapeutic interventions to reduce ICP include osmotic diuretics, controlled hyperventilation, blood pressure control, judicious sedation, head elevation, ventricular CSF drainage, and barbiturate coma.

Osmotic Diuretics

Patients who have clinical signs of herniation or considerable brain swelling on CT should be treated with dehydration therapy if they are hemodynamically stable. Mannitol (0.5 - 1.5 gm/kg body weight) given over 10 minutes reduces ICP. Hyperosmolar agents remove water from normal parts of the brain by creating an osmolar gradient between the blood and areas with an intact blood-brain barrier. The diuretic response is rapid. A Foley catheter should be inserted into the bladder before starting this therapy. The goal is a serum osmolarity of 300 - 310 mOsm/L. Excessive dehydration may result in hypovolemia, acute tubular necrosis, and renal failure.

Blood Pressure Control

The systolic blood pressure should be kept between 100 and 180 mm Hg to optimize cerebral perfusion. The cerebral perfusion pressure is defined as the difference between mean arterial pressure and mean intracranial pressure. The cerebral perfusion pressure should be maintained between 70 and 100 mm Hg, and the ICP should be kept in the normal range (5 - 15 mm Hg). To achieve this goal, there should be close cooperation between the intensive care physician and neurosurgeon.

Elevation of the Head

Keeping the head up 30° to 45° in the midline neutral plane reduces ICP by promoting venous drainage.

Controlled Hyperventilation

During the first 24 hours after a severe brain injury, cerebral blood flow is reduced by more than 50 percent; therefore, controlled hyperventilation should only be employed during the first day if elevated ICP does not respond to dehydration therapy, blood pressure control, and head elevation. Moderate hypocapnia (pCO_2 30 - 35 mm Hg) lowers ICP by vasoconstriction and reduction of cerebral blood flow. Oxygen saturation should be kept above 95 percent, as hypoxia will increase cerebral blood flow.

Seizure Prophylaxis

Prophylaxis with phenytoin is appropriate for preventing seizures within the first seven days of injury. Patients with depressed skull fractures, penetrating injuries, focal neurological deficits, cerebral contusions, or intracranial hemorrhages are at significant risk for seizures (see chapter 8).

Sedation

Sedation and neuromuscular paralysis are often required to maintain full ventilatory support. These medications also prevent spikes in ICP associated with agitation and posturing. Fentanyl is an effective sedative, and an initial bolus of 50 - 100 micrograms can be followed by a continuous infusion. Unlike morphine, fentanyl is not associated with histamine release. Pancuronium or vecuronium may be added to combat excessive muscular activity. Increased ICP, hypoxia, pain and distended bladder are common causes of agitation, and they must be investigated and treated.

Ventricular CSF Drainage

In some patients with acute TBI, intermittment CSF drainage through a ventriculostomy may be an effective means of controlling ICP. With severe TBI, the ventricles are small and compressed, and placement and maintenance of a catheter in the ventricles may be difficult. As a result, ventriculostomy is not a viable option in many people with severe TBI.

Temperature Control

Hyperthermia raises brain metabolism and is associated with a poorer outcome. As such, mild hypothermia of 32°C - 33°C may be beneficial. If the patient has a fever, the cause must be quickly ascertained and appropriate treatment instituted (e.g., antibiotics for a urinary tract infection). Fever should be controlled with acetaminophen or a cooling blanket.

Barbiturate Coma

When the standard therapy outlined above fails to consistently maintain ICP below 25 mm Hg (15 mm Hg in children or in adults with a craniotomy defect), high-dose barbiturate therapy is considered. Sodium pentobarbital and thiopental are the most commonly used barbiturates. A loading dose of 5 - 10 mg/kg is administered over 10 minutes. A precipitous fall in blood pressure can occur if it is given rapidly. A maintenance dose of 3 - 5 mg/kg/hr is given to obtain a serum level of 3 - 5 mg%. Barbiturates should not be used without ICP monitoring. When ICP has been normal for at least 24 hours, barbiturates are withdrawn slowly over 24 to 48 hours to avoid a paradoxical rise in ICP.

Suggested Readings:

Bullock R, Chesnut RM, Clifton G, et al. Guidelines for the management of severe head injury. Brain Trauma Foundation. European Journal of Emergency Medicine 1996; 3(2):109-127.

Narayan RK, Wilberger JE, Povlishock JT, editors. Neurotrauma. New York: McGraw-Hill; 1996.

Ordia JI. Neurologic function seven years after crowbar impalement of the brain. Surgical Neurology 1989; 32:152-155.

Seelig JM, Becker DP, Miller JD, et. al. Traumatic acute subdural hematoma: major mortality reduction in comatose patients treated within four hours. New England Journal of Medicine 1981; 304:1511-1518.

Chapter 4

Initial Rehabilitation Medicine Consultation

Shanker Nesathurai, MD, FRCP(C)
Elizabeth A. Roaf, MD

The purpose of this chapter is to discuss the elements of a physiatric consultation for a traumatic brain injury (TBI) patient. Physiatrists will usually be consulted in the acute hospital for one of two reasons. First, a new TBI patient may be admitted. Second, the patient has a remote injury and is being readmitted for medical problems that may or may not be associated with his TBI. An example of this would be a patient who suffered a TBI remotely and is currently being admitted with aspiration pneumonitis.

With a new injury, the patient may be admitted to the intensive care unit. At this point, the acute medical issues are most important (i.e., appropriate surgical management, management of cerebral edema, fluid resuscitation, etc.). Early physiatric consultation, however, will assist in TBI management and provide an opportunity to educate other members of the health-care team about rehabilitation care. This chapter will focus on the issues that rehabilitation physicians must review in the initial assessment. Many of these topics are discussed in more detail in other chapters.

Elements of a Consultation

There are certain key elements of a consultation. The consultation record should document the name and service of the clinician, as well as the name and service of the individual who requested the consultation. The chart should be thoroughly reviewed, and the pertinent history should be summarized. For a rehabilitation medicine consultation, it is important to document the patient's premorbid vocational and educational status. It is also important to determine the patient's family and home situation. For example, a patient who is financially secure and lives with a caring spouse in a single-floor home has fewer discharge challenges than an unemployed, homeless patient with no family supports.

A thorough history and physical examination are essential. The clinical assessment must include pertinent information, such as duration of loss of consciousness and post-traumatic amnesia and the Glasgow Coma Scale (see overview) score, on admission and at the time of examination. A mental status exam and assessment of the patient's level of recovery as defined by the

Rancho Los Amigos Scale of Cognitive Functioning (see overview) should also be completed. The consultant's recommendations should be legible and easy to understand.

The effective management of TBI requires an understanding of the patient's physical and cognitive impairments. For example, a person with damage to the premotor areas of the frontal lobe may present with impaired gait. This individual may also suffer from uncontrolled episodes of anger and the inability to follow simple commands. To achieve the functional goal of independent mobility, the cognitive and behavioral issues must be addressed to allow for participation in an ambulation training program.

Many times, the rehabilitation team must also educate the family of the injured person. Families may have unrealistic goals or be unable to cope with the change in family dynamics subsequent to a TBI. Some family members may become reluctant caregivers. As such, TBI not only affects the individual, but his family as well.

Comorbid Conditions

Many persons with TBI have co-existing pathology, such as fractures, abdominal wounds, seizure disorders, pneumothoraces, cardiac contusions, and cranial nerve injuries. Some patients also have substance abuse disorders. The consultation record should clearly document these comorbidities, as well as the proposed medical and surgical treatment plan. The rehabilitation treatment plan must include strategies to manage associated impairments, as well as the cognitive sequelae of TBI. On occasion, comorbidity results in a significant adjustment of the rehabilitation plan. For example, a patient with an injury to the dominant hemisphere may benefit from an ambulation program. If this individual has a concomitant acetabular fracture, however, weight bearing may not be permitted for many weeks, and, initially, wheelchair-level goals should be recommended.

Some persons with profound TBI are not able to communicate with their caregivers. On such occasions, additional injuries may not be recognized at the time of initial hospitalization (e.g., unrecognized scaphoid fracture). These injuries may be identified later in the hospitalization. It is imperative that all patients with significant trauma be fully evaluated for concomitant injuries prior to transfer to the rehabilitation unit.

Pressure Ulcers

Many TBI patients have impaired cognition and diminished bed mobility; as such, they are at high risk for skin breakdown. The development of a pressure ulcer can profoundly impact the nature, length and cost of a patient's rehabilitation care. Pressure, shear, maceration and friction will contribute to the development of a skin ulcer. Close skin surveillance is mandatory. Patients should be repositioned every two hours to reduce pressure over vulnerable areas. Extreme care must be used in assisted bed mobility and transfers to minimize friction and shear forces. Excessive perspiration and urinary and fecal incontinence should be treated to minimize maceration. Selected patients, especially those with markedly impaired levels of consciousness, should have a low-air-loss mattress (e.g., Kinair or Clinitron).

Contractures

Immobility can lead to potentially painful contractures, which may diminish function (e.g., gastrocnemius contractures leading to an inability to walk). Muscles that cross two joints, such as the gastrocnemius, hamstrings, iliopsoas and biceps brachii, are at particular risk. Contractures can be prevented by passive range of movement of the joints and proper positioning (e.g., prone lying to minimize iliopsoas contractures). The physical therapy service can assist in contracture prevention. Early ambulation should be encouraged. An ankle foot orthosis can prevent the progression of gastrocnemius contractures. An orthosis, however, is not a substitute for a passive range of movement program (see chapter 11).

Upper Motor Neuron Syndrome and Spasticity

Spasticity is a disorder of muscle tone characterized by a velocity-dependent resistance to passive joint movement. Other manifestations of spasticity include increased muscle stretch reflexes, clonus, and the "clasp-knife" phenomenon. Flexor and cutaneo-motor spasms are common in upper motor neuron diseases. Although these abnormalities are not considered manifestations of spasticity, they may cause significant functional limitations. Spasms can be treated with many of the same management strategies as spasticity.

Spasticity should be treated when it contributes to pain, impairs hygiene, interferes with nursing care, contributes to contractures, or leads to pressure ulcers. Some patients, however, find spasticity helpful with mobility and transfers. As such, the risks and benefits of intervention should be balanced.

Chronic TBI patients who are admitted to the hospital should remain on their spasticity medications. This is particularly important for patients who are on baclofen, since rapid withdrawal can lead to seizures, weakness and mental status changes.

Spasticity can be managed with medications such as dantrolene sodium (Dantrium), tizanidine (Zanaflex), diazepam (Valium), baclofen (Lioresal), and clonidine (Catapres). Other interventions include motor branch blocks, nerve blocks, and botulinum toxin injections. In refractory cases, an intrathecal baclofen pump can be considered (see chapter 9).

DVT Prophylaxis

TBI patients are at very high risk for developing deep venous thrombosis (DVT). Because DVT can lead to a pulmonary embolus and potentially death, prophylaxis is essential. As there is the concern of bleeding at anatomical sites in acute brain injury, anticoagulants are not recommended in the acute phase. At this early stage, mechanical methods of DVT prophylaxis, such as intermittment pneumatic compression devices (e.g., Venodyne boots) and thigh high compression stockings (e.g., TED stockings), are recommended. Some clinicians recommend serial doppler studies. These investigations, however, are expensive and often do not identify a significant number of calf clots.

Minidose subcutaneous unfractionated heparin, adjusted dose subcutaneous unfractionated heparin, or subcutaneous low molecular weight heparin are, however, reasonable interventions later in the course of TBI (perhaps as early as two weeks post-injury). As well, subcutaneous heparin prophylaxis is appropriate for a chronic TBI patient admitted to the hospital for a secondary condition (e.g., skin flap). In patients with a very high risk of DVT and potential pulmonary embolus, such as acute TBI with associated femur and pelvic fractures, a Greenfield filter is indicated.

Pulmonary Issues

Injuries to the central nervous system may impact pulmonary function in a variety of ways. Early after injury, patients with severe head injury may develop neurogenic pulmonary edema. Later in the hospital course, a patient may develop pulmonary embolism, abnormal breathing patterns, and aspiration or nosocomial pneumonia.

Patterns of abnormal breathing during sleep or altered levels of consciousness may be manifested by hypopnea (decreased breathing) or apnea (lack of breathing). Cheyne-Stokes respiration, manifested by a crescendo-descrescendo pattern followed by a brief period of apnea, may occur after injury to the brain. Both of these patterns, as well as altered level of consciousness, may predispose the patient to hypercapnia or, possibly, hypoxemia. Alterations in breathing patterns may be related to focal brain pathology or elevated intracranial pressure (ICP) secondary to hydrocephalus or cerebral swelling. Patients at risk for pulmonary compromise should be intubated and promptly placed on a ventilator. Ventilation will also assist in the management of raised ICP.

Those with a remote TBI may also be at increased risk of developing asymptomatic apnea or hypopnea. Thus, arterial blood gas measurement and overnight oximetry or a sleep study may be needed to fully evaluate this possibility.

Aspiration is frequently a problem in those with traumatic brain injury. Aspiration is associated with a diminished level of consciousness, damage to the cranial nerves, or direct injury to the brain stem. Impaired cough and abnormal ventilatory patterns can also increase the risk of aspiration. If pneumonitis does develop, aggressive chest physical therapy techniques, such as assisted cough, chest wall percussion, postural draining, and frequent suctioning, are indicated. If aspiration pneumonitis becomes a recurrent problem, placement of a percutaneous gastrostomy tube may be needed.

Neuroendocrine Complications

Individuals who have had a traumatic brain injury may suffer from associated neuroendocrine problems due to injury to the posterior or anterior hypothalamus, or both. The syndrome of inappropriate antidiuretic hormone (SIADH) is a common sequela following brain injury. During stressful episodes such as trauma, the hypothalamus increases the release of antidiuretic hormone (ADH), or vasopressin. In TBI, elevated ICP may also further contribute to the release of ADH. The result is an increase in free water absorption in the kidneys and concomitant hyponatremia. Symptoms of SIADH include anorexia, vomiting, weakness, cognitive impairment, headache, agitation and seizures. Profound hyponatremia (less than 100 mEq/L) can be fatal. Patients with TBI may also develop SIADH that is precipitated by medications such as amitriptyline (Elavil), carbamazepine (Tegretol), and phenobarbital.

To diagnose SIADH, measurement of concurrent urinary and serum sodium levels must be undertaken and the fractional excretion of sodium (FENa) must be calculated. The FENa should be greater than 1 percent in SIADH. Characteristically, the urinary sodium is greater than 20 mEq/L and the urine osmolality is greater than 100 mOsm/kg. The diagnosis of SIADH should be made only when renal, adrenal and thyroid function are deemed normal. Panhypopituitarism should also be excluded.

Treatment depends on the severity of hyponatremia or the presence of symptoms. In mild cases (serum sodium greater than 130 mEq/L in an asymptomatic individual), fluid restriction of 1 liter per day should be instituted. With more severe hyponatremia (serum sodium less than 130 mEq/L), or if the patient is symptomatic, he may be treated with normal saline infusion followed by furosemide (Lasix) or bumetadine (Bumex) to avoid fluid overload. In cases of severe hyponatremia (serum sodium less than 120 mEq/L) or in a patient who has developed seizures, the administration of hypertonic saline may be indicated.

If the hyponatremia is corrected too rapidly, the result is central pontine myelinolysis. It is recommended that serum sodium be corrected by no more than 10 to 12 mEq/L in the first 24 hours and no more than 6 mEq/L on subsequent days.

Neurogenic diabetes insipidus (DI) is a less common disorder of the pituitary gland and is associated with basal skull fractures. In this condition, there is diminished vasopressin secretion. It is characterized by an excessive excretion of dilute urine (specific gravity of less than 1.005). Other clinical manifestations include hypernatremia, polyuria, nocturia and polydipsia. The decrease in intravascular volume may lead to hypotension and, thereby, diminish cerebral perfusion pressure. As the condition progresses, a patient may experience mental status changes. If the patient is conscious, increasing oral fluid intake is necessary. If the patient is unconscious, intravenous hypotonic (D5W) fluid replacement must be prescribed. DI can be treated acutely with subcutaneous vasopressin or chronically with nasal desmopressin.

Pain

Patients with traumatic brain injuries may experience significant pain, which may be related to fractures, contusions, muscle spasm, heterotopic ossification, or due to surgical procedures. Headaches are another frequent cause of pain in both acute and chronic head injuries. Peripheral neuropathic pain may also be a concern in those with associated plexopathies or peripheral neuropathies. Pain should be treated with judicious use of narcotic and non-narcotic analgesics. Non-narcotic analgesics should be the first line of management since narcotics may alter mental status in an individual with already compromised cognition. Neurogenic pain may be managed with medications, including carbamazepine (Tegretol), valproic acid (Depakene) gabapentin (Neurontin), clonidine (Catapres), or tricyclic agents (e.g., nortriptyline).

Bowel Management

Most patients with TBI will suffer from constipation. A comprehensive bowel regimen should be instituted. In an acute injury, stool softeners, such as Colace or Senokot, can be started. If possible, the patient should be placed on the commode or bedpan after breakfast to utilize the gastrocolic reflex. If obstipation is suspected, a KUB film should be obtained and a gentle enema can be considered.

Stress gastritis is common after a traumatic injury. The use of a proton pump inhibitor or a histamine-2 blocking agent may be initiated in the early phase after TBI to prevent serious bleeding complications. Abdominal distention, pancreatitis and ileus are possible in the acute phase of injury and may have an atypical presentation due to the patient's potential inability to coherently express his symptoms.

Autonomic Dysfunction

Infrequently, patients with TBI suffer from central dysautonomia. Autonomic disturbances may present with impairments in temperature regulation or with alterations in blood pressure and pulse. "Central fevers" are fevers in which the patient has a high temperature (i.e., above 104° F), but no other findings consistent with infection. This diagnosis should only be made when all other causes of fever have been excluded. Treatment involves cooling the patient, decreasing ambient room temperature, the use of antipyretics, and, possibly, gastric lavage.

If tachycardia and hypertension are associated with high fevers (and the patient does not have asthma), a beta-blocker may help manage the dysautonomia in the acute phase. Acute hydrocephalus has been reported to be associated with central dysautonomic phenomenon.

Nutrition

Adequate nutrition is essential in patients who have suffered multitrauma. Early on during recovery, oral intake may not be possible due to impaired swallowing mechanisms, altered level of consciousness, or multitrauma involving facial structures. Nasogastric or orogastric feeding, followed by the placement of a gastrostomy or jejunostomy tube, may be necessary for adequate nutrition in the early period following the brain injury. As patients begin to show cognitive recovery, a bedside swallowing evaluation followed by a barium swallowing study is reasonable. Although bedside swallowing evaluations are helpful, silent aspiration should be considered in those patients with a history of aspiration, known brain stem or cranial nerve involvement, or dysphagia.

Cognitive Recovery

In this monograph, assessment and treatment are predicated by the assumption that people with TBI recover in a hierarchical manner. In other words, patients progress sequentially through the Rancho Los Amigos Scale of Cognitive Functioning (see overview). Although management strategies must be individualized, there are certain characteristic issues that must be addressed at different levels of recovery. Cognitive recovery can be facilitated by a combination of pharmacological and non-pharmacological interventions. Treatment strategies are discussed further in chapters 5, 6 and 7.

Prognosis

Prognosis in TBI is difficult to predict. Generalizations can be made about populations of patients, but predicting the outcome of a particular patient can be difficult. Caution should be exercised when speaking with family members about prognosis. Better outcomes are associated with Glasgow Coma Scale scores greater than 8, adults between the ages of 25 and 60, post-traumatic amnesia of less than two weeks, and normal neuroimaging. Those individuals diagnosed with diffuse axonal injury may have more functional challenges.

Disposition and Discharge Planning

Discharge planning should begin as soon as the patient is admitted to the hospital. Physiatrists should advocate for appropriate skilled comprehensive TBI care. Institutions with TBI programs certified by the Commission on the Accreditation of Rehabilitation Facilities (CARF) or designated as National Model Traumatic Brain Injury Systems Centers will provide excellent care. Insurance carriers may compel patients to receive rehabilitation services from "preferred" providers. Some patients will request rehabilitation services at sites close to their homes or for other personal reasons.

Long-Term Issues

During the initial consultation, it is important to consider long-term issues. This is particularly true for a patient with a remote TBI. Every patient must be encouraged to locate a primary care physician who is knowledgeable about traumatic brain injury. Health-care services should be available in an architecturally accessible facility. Physiatrists should encourage patients to participate in routine health maintenance (e.g., screening for cancer and cardiovascular disease, as well as updating immunizations, etc.).

Checklist for Acute Traumatic Brain Injury Rehabilitation Medicine Consultation

- Detailed clinical summary of injury
- Document comorbid conditions
- Comprehensive physical examination
- Document initial Glasgow Coma Scale score
- Document current Rancho Los Amigos Scale of Cognitive Functioning level
- Document length of post-traumatic amnesia (if possible)
- Document length of coma

Comment on the Following Issues

- Comorbid conditions
- Pressure ulcers
- Contractures
- Upper motor neuron syndrome and spasticity
- DVT prophylaxis
- Pulmonary issues
- Neuroendocrine complications

- Pain
- Bowel management
- Autonomic dysfunction
- Nutrition
- Cognitive recovery
- Prognosis
- Disposition and discharge planning
- Long-term issues

Suggested Readings:

Kraft GH, Horn LJ. Pharmacology and brain injury rehabilitation. Physical Medicine and Rehabilitation Clinics of North America. Philadelphia: W.B. Saunders; 1997.

Evans RN. Neurology and trauma. Philadelphia: W.B. Saunders; 1996.

Chapter 5

Cognitive Rehabilitation of Traumatic Brain Injury Patients

Lygia Soares, PhD

Cognitive rehabilitation, as stated in the overview of this monograph, encompasses strategies that enhance spontaneous recovery or facilitate compensatory skills following a traumatic brain injury (TBI). It is based on the premise that recovery of function subsequent to a TBI occurs in a hierarchical sequence. Cognitive rehabilitation is the thread that holds the TBI treatment program together; it cannot be successfully executed in isolation. The cognitive treatment plan requires the participation and commitment of the entire team, and must be integrated with the standard physical and medical interventions. To formulate an effective treatment plan, the team must accurately identify a patient's impairments.

Several complementary (and a few mutually exclusive) approaches to cognitive rehabilitation have been proposed over the years. This discussion, however, will focus on interdisciplinary treatment strategies based on impairment as classified by the Rancho Los Amigos Scale of Cognitive Functioning (RLASCF). There is an assumption that recovery will progress in a predictable and recognizable manner. Clearly, this scale cannot reasonably categorize every patient's clinical course. In addition, many patients will not progress through the "stages" of recovery, remaining "fixed" at one Rancho level.

With these caveats noted, patients at the lowest levels of the RLASCF (Levels I, II and III) require a "stimulation" program. At this level of impairment, patients cannot participate in a classic goal-oriented rehabilitation program. The hope of treatment is to "arouse" the patient into a higher level of cognitive function. Level IV is a critical transition phase, as the patient "emerges" from coma, but has episodes of agitation that preclude discipline-specific interventions. As the patient progresses on the continuum of recovery (Levels V and VI), a more structured, goal-oriented approach is necessary. At this point, the patient is more able to participate in a goal-oriented rehabilitation program. At higher levels in the Rancho continuum (Levels VII and VIII), community and vocational integration become more of a focus.

Management of Patients at Levels I, II and III

The common characteristic of patients at Levels I, II and III (No Response, Generalized Response, Localized Response) is diminished interaction with environmental stimuli. A variety of terms have been used to describe programs aimed at treating patients with the highest level of impairment, including "coma arousal therapy, "multisensory therapy," and "coma rehabilitation." The stimulation-oriented approach provides an organized presentation of heightened sensory input with the hope of advancing a patient from his current RLASCF level. Treatment is directed at providing heightened sensory input presented in an organized fashion via all the senses: auditory, visual, olfactory, cutaneous and kinesthetic. Goals of therapy are to prevent sensory deprivation, elicit responses to sensory input, and improve attention.

Important features of a stimulation program should include the following:

- stimuli should be presented in an orderly manner to one input channel at a time
- explanation should be provided prior to the presentation
- treatment sessions should be brief (15 to 20 minutes) but frequent (several times a day) since the patient may fatigue easily and have a limited attention span
- the family should be given the opportunity to participate in the stimulation program.

Common responses to interventions include eye movements, auditory startle, facial grimacing, increased muscle tone, head movements toward or away from the stimuli, withdrawal of limbs to averse stimuli, changes in posturing, and increased respiration. The clinician, however, should not be limited to looking for these responses, but should be aware of any changes in behavior. As treatment progresses, efforts should be directed toward increasing the frequency of occurrence, rate of response, the period of time over which the patient can remain alert, the variety of responses the patient is capable of generating, and the quality of the patient's attention to the environment.

Multisensory stimulation techniques can be provided at the bedside or in a separate treatment area. These interventions can be directed by a variety of disciplines (e.g., physical therapist, occupational therapist, neuropsychologist, speech-language pathologist, etc.). Common treatment strategies include:

- *Visual Stimulation:* Position the patient in an upright position to provide normal visual orientation whenever possible. Use familiar objects, family photographs, or brightly colored objects to work on focusing, tracking and crossing midline. Eliminate distractions to enable the patient to attend visually to the activity. Provide a variety of environments to vary visual input. Television may be used intermittently throughout the day.

- *Auditory Stimulation:* Everyone coming in contact with the patient should be encouraged to speak to the patient. Provide basic orienting information to the patient when working with him. Eliminate extraneous noise to avoid distraction to enable the patient to attend to the auditory stimuli. Use familiar music and tapes provided by family members. Call the patient's name and check for any response and localization of sound. Use loud noises to elicit responses; however, if startle response is consistently elicited, then these stimuli may be detrimental and should not be used. Radio and television may be used intermittently to provide auditory stimulation. If left on too long, however, these sources of stimulation become ambient noise and the patient may stop attending to them.

- *Olfactory Stimulation:* Provide a variety of odors, such as familiar perfumes and colognes, flavorings and assorted spices, and check for any generalizing or localizing response. Noxious odors appear to elicit olfactory responses earlier than other odors. This stimulation modality may be less effective than others as many people with TBI have compromised olfactory pathways. If a tracheostomy is present, the exchange of air through the nose is eliminated, thereby decreasing the olfactory response.

- *Cutaneous Stimulation:* Use a variety of textures, such as fur, feathers, cotton, soft cloths, rubber and sandpaper, to elicit responses. Provide a variety of temperatures, using warm and cold cloths and ice. Vary the degree of pressure when using these different textures. Noxious stimulation, such as pin prick, pinching or squeezing, often elicit the earliest response.

- *Kinesthetic Stimulation:* Place patient on bolsters, bass and rockers to encourage early protective reflexes and delayed balance reactions. Place patient in uncomfortable positions and watch for attempts to reposition himself. Range of motion exercises provide kinesthetic stimulation and give the patient an awareness of his limbs as they are being moved. Bathing and dressing also provide movement of head, trunk and limbs.

- *Oral Stimulation:* Routine mouth care helps in diminishing hypersensitivity, as well as aids in diminishing abnormal oral-facial reflexes. Use of flavored cleansing agents, such as mint or lemon, increases the amount of oral stimulation the patient receives during mouth care. Provide perioral and intraoral stimulation with tongue blades, gloved fingers or ice, and look for relaxation of oral structures. Watch for tactile defensiveness, but continue stimulation to diminish defensive reactions and increase the level of awareness. Early feeding trials can be attempted once all abnormal reflexes are diminished, provided adequate oral control of bolus, swallowing reflex, and cough reflex are present.

As the patient progresses from Level II to Level III, he characteristically localizes to various types of stimulation and may inconsistently follow one-step commands. In these patients, the goal is to increase the frequency, variety, consistency and rate of response, and to expand and channel these responses into simple activities such as hitting a balloon, catching and throwing a large ball, choosing between two objects, matching pictures, and simple self-care tasks.

Neurostimulant medication is sometimes utilized as an adjunct to stimulation-oriented therapy. Pharmacological interventions are discussed in chapter 7.

Management of Patients at Level IV

Patients at Level IV (Confused-Agitated) pose a significant challenge for the treatment team. This is a transition phase, and discipline-specific goals are difficult to establish due to the patient's severely impaired ability to participate in a treatment program. A typical patient at this level is alert but may have episodes of agitation. These outbursts may appear to be signs of regression to an earlier phase. In reality, these potentially troubling behaviors are consistent with the hierarchical progression of recovery. In this phase, the patient cannot be held accountable for his behavior.

Goals of therapy during this stage are to decrease intensity, duration and frequency of agitation and to increase attention to the environment. The team goal is to have the patient progress to a higher cognitive level. The techniques used do not vary significantly among disciplines.

Structure is the foundation of treatment at this level. Since patients at this level have decreased ability to process environmental stimuli, it is imperative that the environment remains constant and non-threatening. The following treatment strategies should be considered:

- the patient must not be left alone unless human contact increases agitation
- unnecessary noise and traffic (i.e., caregivers, housekeeping staff) in the patient's room must be kept to a minimum
- the patient must be oriented frequently with basic information
- physical reassurance must be provided by talking to and touching the patient if he does not object to physical contact
- placing the patient in non-threatening, predictable, highly-structured settings. Initially, the patient might only want to observe the group. Expect participation only when the patient appears comfortable with the group setting
- being sensitive to the patient's tolerance of the activity or group and being prepared to remove the patient or change the activity if restlessness or agitation increase

- removing restraints whenever possible to provide freedom of movement, making sure that the patient is adequately supervised to prevent outbursts

- encouraging participation in simple, automatic self-care tasks like eating, brushing hair or washing face

- sedating psychotropic medication may be used sparingly as a last resort only to prevent the patient from harming himself or others.

Management of Patients at Levels V and VI

Patients at Levels V and VI (Confused-Inappropriate, Confused-Appropriate) continue to demonstrate inappropriate responses to environmental stimuli. Patients demonstrate reduced information processing capacity relative to the amount, rate and duration, and complexity of information provided. People at this level may not be able to perform elementary tasks such as dressing, bathing or feeding. Patients are vulnerable to outside variables and lack the internal mechanism at this point to modulate responses.

Sometimes, reactions to the environment may be exaggerated. For example, prior to injury, a patient may respond to a mildly stressful family situation (e.g., disagreement with spouse about finances) by leaving the room. Subsequent to his TBI, the response may be an exaggerated verbal tirade replete with expletives. Thus, the structure-oriented approach is most effective for use with patients at these levels.

It is at this stage when discipline-specific goals can be established. Tasks must be structured by manipulating the stimulus parameters (i.e., amount, rate, complexity and duration of input). Functional tasks must be simplified into sequential steps. As cognitive capacity increases, structure can be gradually reduced.

Patient Environment

Environment should remain constant in terms of the location of furniture, clothes and personal belongings. Memory aids, such as clocks, calendars and schedules, should be provided within visual range of the patient. Environmental distractions should be minimized. The same nurses and therapists should care for the confused patient every day, if possible. All personnel should provide orienting information at the beginning and end of each interaction.

Speech/Language Pathology Approaches

Language impairment in TBI is a consequence of cognitive dysfunction. Treatment should be directed toward the primary underlying cognitive breakdown, rather than its linguistic consequences. Treatment strategies vary somewhat from Level V to Level VI but essentially focus on increasing attention, orientation, immediate and recent memory, and categorization and sequencing. If other speech or language disturbances are present, the appropriate treatments are begun at these phases of recovery.

Occupational Therapy Approaches

During these stages of recovery, the occupational therapist is able to focus goals on specific areas of deficit such as hygiene, grooming, dressing and self-feeding. In addition, perceptual motor activities, upper extremity exercises, and recreational pursuits should be encouraged. Initially, the activity should be highly structured, but as the patient becomes successful, the structure can be gradually reduced. For example, initially after injury, a patient may require repeated verbal instructions to prepare a simple meal. As the patient progresses, he may simply require supervision to ensure safety with the stove. Still later, the patient may only require a set of written instructions.

Physical Therapy Approaches

The physical therapist also can work on specific goals to improve the patient's motor functioning. Often, occupational and physical therapists work together to improve motor skills, including head control, balance, trunk mobility, strength, range of motion, and mobility. While one therapist gives the verbal or visual directions, the other therapist provides physical support and assistance. As cognition increases, structure is reduced, complexity of task is increased, and verbal cues are reduced. Carry-over learning cannot be expected at this point until memory improves. The physical therapist also assesses equipment needs and provides training in its use, when appropriate.

Home Passes

At Level VI, the family can begin to participate in therapeutic day, overnight or weekend home programs. The familiar surroundings of home usually enhance functional recovery. To ensure a successful home pass, family members should be educated by the treatment team prior to undertaking a pass. Feedback (written and verbal) from families should be solicited by the treatment team with regard to the patient's function during a home visit, and the treatment program should be adjusted accordingly. If the patient is successful for a short time at home and/or cognition improves, then the length of the pass and the demands on the patient are increased. The goal of these passes is to provide continuing structure and prepare the patient and family for a smooth transition to the community upon discharge.

Management of Patients at Levels VII and VIII

The common characteristic of patients at Levels VII and VIII (Automatic-Appropriate, Purposeful-Appropriate) is an automatic response to environmental stimuli. It is transition from dependence to independence, in which people with TBI may be discharged from an institution to a community setting. Patients and families may experience a range of emotions, including anticipation, frustration, anxiety, hope and uncertainty. When patients are discharged from an inpatient setting, it is important that they continue to receive cognitive rehabilitation on an outpatient basis. Although the patient may appear purposeful and goal-directed with minimal confusion in familiar, structured settings, an inability to integrate increased cognitive, physical and emotional skills into meaningful activity becomes apparent as familiarity and structure are decreased. Sometimes these patients may appear to have achieved their premorbid level of cognitive functioning. In reality, many lack the ability to handle stressful situations in social and vocational environments.

As always, the patient's underlying cognitive dysfunction must be taken into account when formulating goals and procedures. As the patient progresses, structural interventions that were required at lower RLASCF levels may become unnecessary. As such, these interventions may, in consultation with the treating clinicians, be gradually withdrawn. For example, a patient who required a memory book at Level V may not require one at Level VII. Alternatively, a patient who required neuropharmacological interventions to manage agitation at Level VI may be able to manage stressful environmental stimuli with behavioral strategies.

Conclusion

Therapy is not only what the clinician does with the patient but also what the patient does with the clinician. Treatment should be focused on changing and modifying a patient's behavior, followed by the generalization of these gains in the community. Thus, in applying the concepts and strategies presented, it is important to keep in mind that cognitive rehabilitation involves teaching a process and not a task.

Successful cognitive rehabilitation requires the concerted effort of physicians, neuropsychologists, nurses, physical and occupational therapists, speech-language pathologists, and the family. Whether pertaining to independence in activities of daily living, communication or cognition, a team effort is necessary to achieve any significant gains.

Suggested Readings:

Malkmus D, Booth B, Kodimer C. Rehabilitation of the head injured adult: comprehensive cognitive management. Downey, CA: Professional Staff Association of Rancho Los Amigos Hospital, Inc.; 1980.

Beukelman D, Yorkston K. Communication disorders following traumatic brain injury: management of cognitive, language, and motor impairment. Austin, TX: Pro Ed; 1991.

Adamovich B, Henderson J, Auerbach S. Cognitive rehabilitation of closed head injured patients: a dynamic approach. Boston: College Hill Press, Inc.; 1985.

Chapter 6

Neuropsychological Interventions for Moderate to Severe Traumatic Brain Injury Patients

Buck H. Woo, PhD

Neuropsychologists working within the rehabilitation setting with traumatic brain injury (TBI) patients focus on three main objectives. First, the neuropsychologist must perform an assessment and construct a neuropsychological profile of the brain injured patient. Second, the neuropsychologist helps to guide the patient's treatment team in areas related to cognitive, behavioral and emotional disorders. Finally, the neuropsychologist provides direct treatment through individual, group and family psychotherapy, or by developing cognitive and behavioral treatment plans with the interdisciplinary rehabilitation team.

It is beyond the scope of this chapter to provide a comprehensive review of neuropsychological techniques and interventions. Instead, this chapter outlines the role of the rehabilitation neuropsychologist in the treatment of people with TBI.

The Approach

Neuropsychological assessment and treatment of persons who have sustained acute TBI are not static events. This is because the cognitive, emotional and behavioral problems TBI patients manifest are considered part of a dynamic process. TBI patients must be followed serially to accurately ascertain the pattern of cognitive recovery and adjust treatment accordingly. Neuropsychologists treating severely impaired brain injured patients must rely on a "process-oriented" approach that demands knowledge of TBI recovery, as well as flexibility in the assessment of methods and instruments that are used. An alternative "fixed battery" approach, which focuses heavily on the administration of standardized tests, is too restrictive to successfully assess patients who have continuously evolving physical and cognitive impairments.

Many neuropsychological instruments may be used to obtain a quantifiable score, as well as more qualitative and process-oriented data. For example, the Rey-Osterreith Complex Figure Test can yield standardized scores on visual-spatial accuracy and visual-spatial memory for comparisons with normal populations in the U.S. (Figures 6.1a, 6.1b and 6.1c). This test also allows the clinician the opportunity to judge planning, organization and problem solving skills by observing the "process" the patient uses to perform this task. Thus, the neuropsychologist must rely on observation, modifiable clinical instruments (tests), and interdisciplinary team and family reports.

Neuropsychological Assessment and Profile

The recognition and classification of a TBI can be a challenge. Often-times patients will not show signs of traumatic brain injury on their neuroimaging studies during the initial acute phase of their hospitalization. A negative CT or MRI study does not exclude a TBI. In addition, patients may be heavily sedated during the acute phase of their treatment, masking underlying signs of TBI (i.e., cognitive, emotional and behavioral abnormalities). Since early detection and treatment of TBI may be associated with better functional outcomes, it is important to provide neuropsychological services to all appropriate patients.

A neuropsychological assessment includes a thorough review of the history and medical records. Important points to note include loss of consciousness, changes in mentation, alterations in behavior (e.g., combativeness), and a history of prior TBI. Other important elements include premorbid intellectual, educational and social status. It is also important to ascertain any history of substance abuse and to document the patient's drug profile and medical comorbidity. Many co-existing medical conditions can impair cognition, including anemia, uremia and sepsis. Medications, such as sedatives, anticonvulsants, narcotics and steroids, can also impair cognitive function. Although imperfect, the patient's clinical status should be classified by the Glasgow Coma Scale and the Rancho Los Amigos Scale of Cognitive Functioning (see overview).

The next step is developing a neuropsychological profile of the patient's cognitive and emotional functioning. This profile should be easily understood by all team members and should not contain unnecessary jargon. This assessment is done serially and frequently since an acutely injured TBI patient's status can change rapidly.

The neuropsychological profile provides a foundation for the rehabilitation team to form its treatment strategies. TBI patients vary considerably in their specific presentation within different stages of recovery. The neuropsychological profile should provide the treatment team with an accurate account of the patient's cognitive and emotional strengths and weaknesses. This will assist the treatment team in developing an effective individualized

Rey-Osterreith Complex Figure Test of a 25-Year-Old Male with Bilateral Frontal Contusions and Traumatic Subarachnoid Hemorrhage

6.1a.

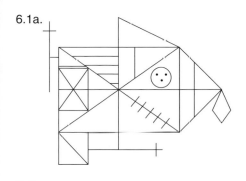

6.1a-Test Stimulus: a patient is asked to reproduce a standardized figure.

6.1b.

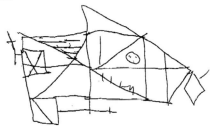

6.1b-With the original figure available, the patient drawing demonstrates impairment of detail and proportion consistent with visual-spatial dysfunction.

6.1c.

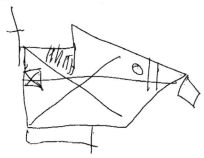

6.1c-The patient is asked to reproduce the figure 30 minutes after initial presentation. The figure must be reproduced from memory. Impairment of visual-spatial memory is clearly demonstrated.

treatment program to take advantage of the patient's unique pattern of cognitive functioning. For example, some patients at Rancho Los Amigos Scale of Cognitive Functioning (RLASCF) Level IV, despite being agitated and confused, may still have enough preservation of language and procedural memory functions to be able to perform simple one- or two-step tasks and engage in "automatic" activities (e.g., holding a pen, drinking from a cup). Therefore, once discovered, these areas of relative strength will form the initial foundation for participation in an acute rehabilitation program.

Neuropsychological Areas to be Assessed

There are six essential areas of cognition that must be assessed in patients who have sustained moderate to severe TBI: attention, memory, language, visual-spatial and executive functions, and personality (emotional/behavioral) functions.

Attention can be defined as the patient's ability to receive and initially process stimuli from the environment. Attention deficits are associated with diffuse brain injuries and are particularly known to occur in patients with frontal lobe pathology. Moreover, deficits in attention will have a significant effect on other areas of cognitive performance, including memory and language comprehension.

Attention can be assessed informally during the course of the evaluation by observing how well patients are able to concentrate on questions and tasks posed to them. It is also important to observe the ease by which they are distracted by external stimuli, such as hallway noise. Attention can be measured more formally using "automatic" tasks, which have few practice effects. These include counting backward from 20 to one, reciting the alphabet, or counting forward by threes. Sustained attention can be measured by using structured tasks, which require longer periods of concentration.

Memory is the cornerstone of successful neuropsychological rehabilitation. Indeed, memory dysfunction is a major limiting factor in successful brain injury rehabilitation. There are many classifications used to describe memory. For the purposes of this discussion, two types of memory will be distinguished: declarative memory and procedural memory.

Declarative memory is a term used to describe facts and events that are directly accessible to conscious recollection. This includes remembering phone and Social Security numbers, addresses, or a list of items to be bought at the supermarket. Declarative memory can be measured when a standardized test of memory is administered.

Procedural memory takes place outside of consciousness. Procedural memory is embedded within learned skills, habits and modifiable cognitive operations. This includes the ability to drive a car or perform most routine activities of daily living (e.g., dressing, bathing and dining).

These two separate memory systems are often affected very differently after a traumatic brain injury. For example, an acute brain injured patient may perform poorly on a task of declarative memory, such as learning a list of new words. The same patient, however, will be able to learn to use the bathroom to toilet and bathe in a new hospital environment. It is important to note that while declarative memory is eventually important during rehabilitation, a brain injury patient may make a successful start in his rehabilitation with relative sparing of procedural memory alone.

There are numerous standardized memory tests available to measure declarative memory (e.g., Weschler Memory Scale III Word List Test, Rey Auditory Verbal Learning Test, California Verbal Learning Test, Benton Visual Retention Test). In contrast, procedural memory is assessed by observing the patient performing activities, including bathing, dressing or dining, and learning modifications to previously well-learned skills to compensate for new physical impairments.

Language is complex and can be difficult to assess. For the purposes of assessing acute TBI, one must focus on an evaluation of the patient's basic comprehension, expression and repetition. Initially, at RLASCF Levels II through IV, simple comprehension assessments can be made by having the patient follow verbal and written commands. More complex comprehension evaluations can be made as the patient progresses through Levels VI and VII, which involve tasks that require greater degrees of information processing (e.g., asking "Does a cork sink in water?"). Expression tasks include confrontational naming in which patients are asked to name common objects presented to them, as well as sentence writing and verbal expression. Repetition is tested by simply having the patient repeat common words and then adding words that occur with less frequency in general everyday use.

Visual-spatial abilities can be assessed by having the patient attempt to copy unique figures. If physical impairments prevent this, tasks requiring the patient to manipulate blocks to copy patterns may be used.

Executive functions involve the patient's ability to organize, plan and execute purposeful behaviors. Self-regulation is an important aspect of executive functions and encompasses the patient's ability to be aware of his behavior and to restrict or express his impulses or desires as appropriate. For example, a patient who continually tries to get out of bed despite restrictions, while verbally acknowledging the safety issues, demonstrates a deficit in executive functions. Self-regulation is also responsible for the modulation of affect and production of socially appropriate conduct. Thus, a deficit in self-regulation is suspected when patients are observed to be disinhibited or emotionally labile. Executive functions can be evaluated at the bedside by observing the appearance of these behaviors throughout the clinical examination. Other deficits in this domain can be elicited by presenting tasks demanding initiation, sequencing, and having the ability to switch easily between tasks (cognitive flexibility).

Personality evaluation refers to the assessment of emotional and behavioral changes that may have occurred due to the TBI. In order to perform a personality evaluation, a careful history must be obtained from family members and others who knew the patient prior to the brain injury.

Cognitive Disorders and Behavioral Syndromes Due to TBI

Specific post-TBI cognitive deficits and behavioral syndromes are often associated with selectively injured areas of the brain. Cognitive and behavioral disorders, however, vary greatly following TBI due to complex neuronal interconnections. Despite this, knowledge of the most commonly discussed cognitive disorders and behavioral syndromes associated with neuroanatomical injury can serve as a common point of reference for neuropsychologists with other TBI clinicians. Thus, a brief review of common disorders associated with the frontal, parietal, temporal and occipital lobes is provided.

Frontal lobe disorders are consistent with impairments of insight, judgment, logical reasoning, memory and problem solving. In addition, executive functions deficits are common. The term "frontal lobe syndrome" for TBI patients refers to behavioral disorders associated with injuries to this area of the brain. There are two major subtypes of frontal lobe syndromes: convexity syndrome and orbitalmedial syndrome. Convexity syndrome is believed to be produced by lesions of or near the lateral surface of the frontal lobe and is associated with apathy, indifference and behavioral withdrawal. Orbitalmedial syndrome is distinguished by a wider variety of manifestations, ranging from behavioral withdrawal to manic types of intense and labile affect, mood swings, impulsiveness and confabulation.

Parietal lobe disorders are associated with agnosia (inability to recognize sensory stimuli), apraxia (inability to perform purposeful movements), and aphasia (language disorder). Lesions of the nondominant hemisphere are associated with a loss of awareness of one's own deficits (anosognosia) and constructional apraxia (inability to reproduce simple patterns or objects). Patients with parietal lobe dysfunction also manifest visual-spatial disorders and hemispatial neglect. Patients with injuries to the dominant hemisphere may present with a variety of language and speech disorders. Common affective changes include apathy, indifference and depression.

Temporal lobe disorders are commonly characterized by disturbances of affect, behavior and cognition that occur with or without accompanying seizures. Patients usually exhibit significant short-term memory disorders. Affective manifestations include severe anxiety, depression, rage or fear. Patient's may also manifest a fluent aphasia (speech lacking in content), alexia (inability to read), and agraphia (inability to express thoughts in writing) with lesions of the dominant hemisphere.

Occipital lobe disorders are hallmarked by visual disturbances. These include an inability to attend to more than one stimulus at a time in a visual field (visual inattention). A person's inability to realize his blindness, to the extent he acts as though sighted, is also associated with injury to the occipital lobe (i.e., occipital blindness).

Treatment

In addition to assessing TBI patients, rehabilitation neuropsychologists are also involved in direct patient treatment. This includes coordinating rehabilitation services, developing behavioral treatment plans, and providing individual, group and family psychotherapies. Neuropsychologists also monitor the effectiveness of drug therapies.

Cognitive rehabilitation includes strategies that enhance spontaneous recovery or facilitate compensatory skills following a TBI. It is best conceptualized as a team function, with all members of the treatment team contributing to an overall cognitive rehabilitation treatment plan.

Behavioral therapy is a form of treatment used to modify a TBI patient's behavior by manipulating environmental events. Behavioral therapy is dependent on identifying behaviors clinicians wish to influence (target behaviors), the triggering (antecedent) events, and providing stimuli (reinforcement) that will reward desired behaviors and diminish unwanted behaviors. The behavioral plan is best developed by the entire treatment team and, if possible, with patient consent and family involvement.

Psychotherapy refers to "talk" therapies that fall into many schools of practice (e.g., supportive therapy, psychoanalytic therapy). TBI patients who would benefit from this therapy must have some degree of insight into their behaviors and be able to utilize certain amounts of judgment, reasoning and problem solving. Thus, this type of therapy is more suitable for mild TBI patients or patients who have progressed to at least RLASCF Level VI.

Suggested Readings:

Lezak MD. Neuropsychological assessment. 3rd ed. New York: Oxford University Press; 1995.

Hanson S, Tucker D. Neuropsychological assessment: physical medicine and rehabilitation — state of the art reviews. Philadelphia, PA: Hanley & Belfus, Inc.; 1992.

Ashley M, Krych D. Traumatic brain injury rehabilitation. Boca Raton, FL: CRC Press; 1995.

Chapter 7

Neuropharmacology After Traumatic Brain Injury

Mark Kaplan, MD

Neuropharmacologic agents are used in traumatic brain injury (TBI) to enhance cognitive function, treat emotional disorders, and minimize behavior dysfunction. By managing these impairments, functional abilities may improve. The utilization of neuropharmacologic agents with TBI patients is a relatively primitive science, and it is important to acknowledge their limitations when used alone. Foremost among these is that cognition is not an isolated or simple function of the central nervous system, but rather a complex integration of neural connections and systems. This complexity is the result of millions of years of evolution of the mammalian brain and, for each individual, years of development and learning. Currently, medications cannot substitute for this complexity, nor are there medications that can repair or regenerate specific neural systems. For example, there is no medication designed specifically for improving insight, judgment, learning or planning. Instead, medications influence neurotransmitters that are widely spread throughout the brain; this influence may secondarily alter and improve an individual's cognition and functional performance. Thus, neuropharmacologic agents are rarely used as the only treatment for a TBI patient. Instead, neuropharmacologic agents are most effective when integrated into a comprehensive cognitive rehabilitation program.

Protocol for the Use of Neuropharmacologic Agents

Optimize conditions

As a general rule, the patient's medical condition should be optimized before starting a neuropharmacologic agent. A patient with an unrecognized urinary tract infection or painful musculoskeletal injury may have a significant "internal" stimulus which, when treated, may allow the patient to refocus his attention on external stimuli, leading to improvements in cognitive functioning. If a neuropharmacologic medication is added at approximately the same time, it will be difficult to separate the effects of the medication from the change in the patient's medical condition.

Review the patient's medications and, if possible, eliminate or reduce the dose of those with potential adverse cognitive side effects. Often, patients improve medically or cognitively and medications that were necessary at one point in the individual's care may be continued unnecessarily. For example, a patient may be receiving unnecessary prophylactic treatment for seizures. If continued treatment is necessary, substitute medications with less potential for adverse cognitive impact. For example, carbamazepine, phenytoin and phenobarbital have some effects on cerebral function. Studies suggest, however, that, of the three medications, carbamazepine has fewer cognitive side effects (see chapter 8).

Identify the target behaviors and contributing variables

In order to utilize neuropharmacologic medications effectively, one must first identify target behaviors and the variables that are affecting them. After this is done, the treatment team must decide on the most appropriate cognitive, behavioral, and neuropharmacologic treatments. This interdisciplinary approach is important since each target behavior is likely to have several cognitive and/or emotional variables contributing to it. For example, one functional target behavior may be dressing skills. The patient's inability to dress himself may be due to a combination of poor sustained attention and disinhibited behaviors. If one uses a neurostimulant medication alone, the patient's attention may improve, but his disinhibition may increase and negate any gains that could have been made. Thus, the use of neuropharmacologic agents must be carefully evaluated and specific variables contributing to the behaviors fully identified. Once this has occurred the team can design a treatment plan to which neuropharmacologic agents can lend valuable support. For example, a neurostimulant to improve attention may be used with a behavioral modification program that reduces disinhibited behaviors to help a patient improve independence in dressing.

Find measures that establish a baseline

It is important to have some way of evaluating the effectiveness of the neuropharmacologic agents that are prescribed. It is recommended that data be gathered from the patient, therapists and family to fully appreciate the effectiveness of the medication. Gathering data from different sources reduces the possibility that a single variable will misrepresent the effectiveness of the neuropharmacologic agent. The ideal measures are objective, specific to the process and individual being measured, and have no practice effects. For example, Ritalin can be prescribed to improve attention, memory and psychomotor speed. A test of digit span can be used to discretely measure attention and immediate memory. In addition, the patient's therapists can report on functional tasks that require sustained attention (e.g., cooking a meal). Meanwhile, when they visit, family members may give input as to whether they believe the patient's memory has improved.

Choose a neuropharmacologic agent

Choosing a neuropharmacologic agent is based on identification of the target behaviors to be modified and understanding the variables influencing the target behaviors. Identifying and treating the target behaviors with neuropharmacologic medications can be a difficult process. The results of a cognitive assessment are important. Other considerations are the onset of action and potential side effects of a medication. One should be cautious about using an agent that would interact in opposition to a medication that the patient is currently taking. For example, a patient receiving a dopamine antagonist (e.g., haloperidol) should not be prescribed a dopamine agonist concomitantly. Also, consider a medication with potentially desirable side effects. For example, a patient with hypertension might benefit from the antihypertensive effects of bromocriptine. A patient with abulia and a Parkinsonian-like movement disorder might be started on Sinemet. A list of frequently used medications for TBI patients is listed in Table 1.

Start the medication and adjust the dose

Medications should be started at the manufacturer's recommended initial dose, with close monitoring for potential side effects. If the patient tolerates the medication, the dose can be titrated upward until either a therapeutic effect is achieved or untoward side effects occur.

Repeat the measures

As the medication is started and the dose adjusted, repeat the baseline functional, psychometric and subjective measures. If a medication is found to be helpful, consider increasing the dose. Another agent that affects the same neurotransmitter but works by a different mechanism might be added. Also, consider adding other medications that affect different transmitters, repeating the steps for dosing as described above.

Consider trials off of the neuropharmacologic agent

Abruptly discontinuing a medication may offer the best opportunity to assess efficacy. This may occur if the patient stops taking the medication or if the prescription inadvertently runs out. On the other hand, the abrupt withdrawal of a medication may, in itself, lead to a decline in cognitive function; therefore, a gradual reduction may be preferred.

Table 1
**Medications in the Management
of Traumatic Brain Injury**

Generic Name	Brand Name	Indications	Starting Oral Dose	Maximum Dose	Common Side Effects
amantadine	Symmetrel	inattention hypo-arousal abulia	100 mg bid	300 mg/day	nausea, dizziness, insomnia
bromocriptine	Parlodel	inattention neglect hypo-arousal abulia	1.25 - 2.5 mg bid	100 mg/day	hypotension, confusion, nausea, dizziness, Raynaud's Phenomenon
buspirone	BuSpar	anxiety agitation	7.5 mg bid	60 mg/day	dizziness, nausea, headache, nervousness
carbamazepine	Tegretol	agitation seizures aggression	200 mg bid	2400 mg/day	rash, photosensitivity, GI upset, dizziness
carbidopa/ levodopa	Sinemet	inattention hypo-arousal abulia	1 tablet (25 mg/ 100 mg) bid–qid	8 tablets/day	GI upset, dizziness
doxepin	Sinequan	insomnia depression	75 mg qhs	300 mg/day	drowsiness, anticholinergic effects, weight gain
haloperidol	Haldol	agitation severe aggression psychosis	1-5 mg bid or tid	100 mg/day	drowsiness, seizures, hypotension, extrapyramidal symptoms
methylphenidate	Ritalin	inattention hypo-arousal abulia	5 mg bid	60 mg/day	insomnia, hypertension, anorexia, anxiety, akathisia

nortriptyline	Pamelor	depression inattention arousal	25 mg qhs	150 mg/day	sedation, anticholinergic effects, lowering of seizure threshold
propranolol	Inderal	agitation aggression	40 mg bid	640 mg/day	dizziness, fatigue, bradycardia, hypotension
protriptyline	Vivactil	inattention hypo-arousal abulia	10 mg qd	60 mg/day	sedation, anticholinergic effects, lowering of seizure threshold
risperidone	Risperdal	agitation inattention hypo-arousal abulia	0.5-1 mg bid	10 mg/day	anxiety, sedation, extrapyramidal symptoms
sertraline	Zoloft	depression	25-50 mg qd	200 mg/day	GI upset, insomnia, drowsiness
trazodone	Desyrel	insomnia depression	50 mg qhs	600 mg/day	drowsiness, seizures, anticholinergic effects, priapism in males (rare)
valproic acid	Depakene	mood swings agitation	250 mg tid	4200 mg/day	changes in menstrual cycle, fatigue, nausea, vomiting, diarrhea, abdominal cramps, anorexia, thrombocytopenia, hepatic failure

Pharmacologic Treatment of Cognitive Disorders

There are very few controlled studies regarding pharmacologic enhancement of cognitive functions after TBI. Moreover, there is a limited amount of cognitive enhancing agents to treat TBI. A brief review is offered of three frequently prescribed neurostimulants. A larger variety of medications is reviewed in Table 1.

Methylphenidate

Methylphenidate is an indirect catecholamine agonist that is a frequently used neurostimulant with cognition-enhancing properties. It has been linked to improvement in learning and memory functions in TBI patients. Studies also support its use in improving attention and distractibility. In fact, methylphenidate is useful in treating agitation associated with impairments in attention following TBI. The short half-life of methylphenidate, however, necessitates two to four doses per day.

Amantadine

Amantadine is a dopaminergic agent. It is a well-tolerated drug that has been successfully used in the treatment of several cognitive disorders following TBI. Amantadine may improve visual attention, speed of information processing, and concentration. It has also be shown to assist in the recovery of patients who are under-responsive or have problems with distractibility.

Bromocriptine

Bromocriptine is a dopamine agonist. It is effective in managing several disorders associated with frontal lobe mediated cognitive functioning, including verbal learning, procedural memory, and hemispatial neglect syndromes.

Treatment of Acute Affective Disorders

Agitation

Agitation and associated aggressive and assaultive behaviors represent some of the most challenging problems for treatment providers and families. Because agitation associated with TBI recovery is usually a self-limiting phenomenon, no pharmacologic intervention may be indicated. Instead, behavioral interventions combined with a structured low-stimulus environment (see chapter 5) may be the most appropriate intervention over this short period.

Benzodiazepines and anti-psychotic medications are not considered first-line medications in the treatment of agitation because of their negative impact on neurologic recovery following TBI. They are recommended, however, at times when a patient poses an immediate danger to himself or severely interferes with life-saving medical care. Low doses of anti-psychotic medications used sparingly, such as haloperidol (Haldol) or risperidone (Risperdal), may have less impact on cognitive recovery than benzodiazepines.

Buspirone (BuSpar) is an anxiolytic agent that is chemically unrelated to benzodiazepines and may decrease agitation in TBI patients. Unlike benzodiazepines, buspirone does not impair cognitive recovery in TBI patients.

Beta-blockers, such as propranolol, may reduce agitation associated with sympathic hyperarousal. Anti-seizure medications, such as carbamazepine and valproic acid, may be helpful for treating patients with episodic behavioral dyscontrol and/or mood swings following TBI.

Neurostimulants, including methylphenidate and amantadine, have been utilized successfully in reducing agitation associated with deficits in attention and distractibility. By increasing attention, the patient is believed to be calmed by improving his awareness of the environment.

Anxiety

Anxiety associated with TBI may manifest as restlessness, poor endurance, decreased concentration, and irritability. As mentioned earlier, benzodiazepines are not recommended because of their negative effects on acute cognitive recovery. In addition, chronic use of benzodiazepines carries risks of physical dependence. Buspirone may be an effective anxiolytic for some patients. It is recommended because it does not negatively affect cognitive recovery. In addition, tricyclic antidepressants can effectively reduce anxiety and may have anti-panic effects. Some commonly prescribed agents include amitriptyline, nortriptyline and doxepin. Beta-blockers, such as propranolol, have also been successfully used to control anxiety in TBI patients.

Depression

Depression is reported to frequently occur among patients who have suffered a TBI. The prevalence of depression following TBI is reported to range from 10 percent to 60 percent. Several antidepressant medications have been shown to be effective for depressed TBI patients. Selective serotonin reuptake inhibitors (SSRI), such as sertraline (Zoloft), and tricyclic antidepressant medications, including despiramine and protriptyline, may be helpful. Protriptyline can be helpful in depressed patients who also have impairment of arousal and/or initiation.

Conclusion

The use of neuropharmacologic agents to enhance TBI recovery requires a systematic approach, as well as clinical experience. TBI is not a single entity. Its neuropathology produces a wide variety of cognitive and behavioral disturbances, and only a few of these manifestations fall into clinically identifiable syndromes (see chapter 6). Moreover, neuropharmacologic agents will have different effects, depending on the patient's physiological injuries, stage of recovery, and personal history. There are very few controlled studies for the use of neuropharmacologic agents with TBI patients. Therefore, rehabilitation physicians must use astute clinical observation, experience, and case studies to guide their treatment decisions.

Suggested Readings:

Ashley M, Krych D. Traumatic brain injury rehabilitation. Boca Raton, FL: CRC Press, 1995.

Barrett AM, Crucian GP, Schwartz RL, Heilman KM. Adverse effect of dopamine agonist therapy in a patient with motor-intentional neglect. Archives of Physical Medicine & Rehabilitation 1999 May; 80(5):600-3.

Feeney DM. From laboratory to clinic: noradrenergic enhancement of physical therapy for stroke or trauma patients. Advances in Neurology 1997; 73:383-94.

Glenn MB. Methylphenidate for cognitive and behavioral dysfunction after traumatic brain injury. Journal of Head Trauma Rehabilitation 1998 Oct; 3(5):87-90.

Gualtieri CT, Evans RW. Stimulant treatment for the neurobehavioral sequelae of traumatic brain injury. Brain Injury 1998 Oct-Dec; 2(4):273-90.

Gualtieri CT. Pharmacotherapy and the neurobehavioral sequelae of traumatic brain injury. Brain Injury 1998 Apr-Jun: 2(2):101-29.

Hornstein A, Lennihan L, Seliger G, Lichtman S, Schroeder K. Amphetamine in recovery from brain injury. Brain Injury 1996 Feb; 10(2):145-8.

Hurford P, Stringer AY, Jann B. Neuropharmacologic treatment of hemineglect: a case report comparing bromocriptine and methylphenidate. Archives of Physical Medicine & Rehabilitation 1998 Mar; 79(3): 346-9.

Kraus MF. Neuropsychiatric sequelae of stroke and traumatic brain injury: the role of psychostimulants. International Journal of Psychiatry in Medicine 1995; 25(1):39-51.

Rizzo M, Tranel. Head injury and postconcussive syndrome. New York: Churchill Livingstone; 1996.

Wroblewski B, Glenn MB, Cornblatt R, Joseph AB, Suduikis S. Protriptyline as an alternative stimulant medication in patients with brain injury: a series of case reports. Brain Injury 1993 Jul-Aug; 7(4);353-62.

Chapter 8

Management of Post-Traumatic Seizure Disorders

David Burke, MD, MA
Anantha Kamath, MD

People with traumatic brain injuries (TBI) have a twelve-fold increase in the incidence of seizures. While much of the information on seizure activity after brain injury has come from military literature, some information is now available concerning the occurrence of post-TBI seizures in civilian populations. A recent population-based study determined the incidence of seizures subsequent to mild, moderate and severe TBI to be 1.5 percent, 2.9 percent, and 17 percent, respectively. The incidence of post-traumatic seizures is related to the severity of the brain injury (i.e., patients with severe TBI are more likely to have seizures than mild TBI patients).

Prominent factors (the first three are the most significant high-risk combination of factors) that are found to be associated with an increased risk for post-traumatic seizures include:

- CT-documented "extended cortical lesions" (i.e., cortical lesions with subcortical extensions)
- depressed skull fractures
- prolonged post-traumatic amnesia
- missile injuries with dural penetration and retained metal fragments
- intracerebral hemorrhage
- diffuse brain contusion
- loss of consciousness for more than 24 hours
- focal neurological signs on the initial examination
- frontal lesions
- advanced age
- recreational drug use.

Post-traumatic seizures can be divided into immediate (within hours of injury), early (within the first week of injury), and late (one week or more post-injury) seizures. Most patients who have seizures will have an initial event within the first two years subsequent to injury; however, about 12 percent to 15 percent of patients will have their first unprovoked seizure 10 to 30 years after severe TBI.

Pohlmann-Eden has reported the distribution of post-traumatic seizures as one-quarter exclusively partial, one-quarter essentially generalized, and one-half combined partial with secondarily generalized seizures. Generalized tonic-clonic seizures typically include a clear and sudden loss of consciousness, followed by tonic extension of the arms and legs, then clonic rhythmic limb jerking, and ultimately ending with flaccidity, stupor and labored deep breathing. Incontinence is usually present. Partial seizures usually result from localized involvement of any part of the motor or sensory cortex and are always associated with retention of consciousness. Examples include single limb jerks; visual aura (e.g., spots, lights, geometric shapes); auditory symptoms (e.g., ringing, buzzing, clicking sounds); unpleasant tastes or smells; and localized numbness. Occasionally, partial seizures may be characterized by other autonomic, visceral, psychic, sensory or motor symptoms, including posturing of the head and eyes, slow repetitive limb movements, fluctuating heart rate, flushing, lip smacking, and arm fidgeting. These may often be clinically difficult to recognize as seizure phenomena.

Seizure Prophylaxis

Early post-traumatic seizures may negatively affect recovery from TBI by increasing brain metabolic demands and elevating intracranial pressure. A seizure may also cause excessive neurotransmitter release. Although this hypothesis has not been convincingly demonstrated in epidemiological or animal studies, many clinicians advocate for seizure prophylaxis. Temkin and colleagues, however, have shown that prophylactic treatment with phenytoin will only result in reduced incidence of seizures in the first week post-injury. Although patients with moderate or severe TBI would probably benefit from prophylaxis, patients with insignificant TBI (i.e., mild TBI with no other risk factors) would probably not.

Ordering anti-seizure medications beyond one week is not recommended, unless the patient has had a documented seizure in the hospital or is at very high risk for seizures (e.g., missile wound with significant tissue loss, history of seizures prior to TBI, etc.). It should be remembered, however, that phenytoin provides no protective effect against the development of late post-traumatic seizures.

Treating Documented Seizures

The diagnosis of a seizure disorder in TBI patients can be a challenge. In severely injured, comatose patients, seizure activity may not be readily recognized as a seizure. An EEG can be helpful in determining if a patient's clinical presentation is consistent with a seizure disorder. On occasion, an ambulatory 24- or 48-hour EEG is indicated.

In general, if a patient has had a seizure subsequent to TBI, anti-convulsant treatment is warranted. One area of controversy, however, is a seizure within 24 hours of injury. These individuals may not require long-term treatment with anti-seizure medications.

Medications that are indicated for treatment include phenytoin, carbamazepine, valproic acid and gabapentin (see Table 1). The type of seizure should determine long-term medication selection. Medication choice, however, should be tempered by the potential cognitive and non-cognitive side effects. Anti-seizure medications may impair the natural progress of neuronal recovery. Although not universally accepted, some argue that anti-seizure medications may adversely impact brain plasticity, diminish learning, and depress cognitive recovery. Some agents have more profound cognitive side effects than others. For example, carbamazepine is putatively believed to have fewer side effects than phenytoin. Thus, if both medications are deemed equally efficacious for a particular type of seizure, then carbamazepine may be the preferred agent.

The exact duration of treatment is arbitrary. If a patient remains seizure-free for two years, one can reasonably consider withdrawing anti-seizure medications. Because available data does not indicate that long-term treatment is beneficial toward preventing post-traumatic seizures, some physicians prefer tapering as early as six months. One-third of people with the first episode of seizures after one week (i.e., late seizures) subsequent to a TBI will have a recurrence after the withdrawal of anti-seizure medications. Discontinuing the medication may have implications for driving an automobile and perhaps returning to work (e.g., operating a forklift or crane). Some clinicians recommend that patients refrain from driving while anti-seizure medications are weaned. The practice of discontinuing anti-seizure medications on the basis of an EEG is not recommended. The presence of abnormalities on an EEG does not always correlate with future seizure risk.

Table 1
Anti-Seizure Medications

Medication	phenytoin	carbamazepine	valproic acid	gabapentin
Brand Name	Dilantin	Tegretol	Depakene	Neurontin
Mechanism of Action	stabilizes neuronal membranes and decreases seizures by changing membrane permeability to sodium ions	depresses activity leading to neuronal discharge by limiting the influx of sodium ions across cell membranes	increases GABA's inhibitory effects	unknown; structurally related to GABA, but does not bind to GABA receptors
Starting Oral Dose	Load 15-20 mg/kg in 3 divided doses every 2-4 hours to increase absorption Maintenance 5-6 mg/kg/day in 3 divided doses	200 mg bid (increase by 200 mg/day at weekly intervals until desired effect is reached)	10-15 mg/kg/day in 3 divided doses (increase by 5-10 mg/kg/day at weekly intervals until desired effect is reached)	day 1 - 300 mg qhs day 2 - 300 mg bid day 3 - 300 mg tid
Maximum Oral Dose	1,500 mg over 24 hours (loading)	2,400 mg/day	4,200 mg/day	1,800 mg/day
Therapeutic Range	10-20 ug/ml	6-12 ug/ml	50-100 ug/ml	routine monitoring not required
Special Considerations	therapeutic level must be adjusted for low albumin	caution with cardiac or hepatic diseases	monitor LFTs, CBCs and platelets	abrupt withdrawal may precipitate seizures
Common Side Effects	IV effects, hypotension, bradycardia, cardiac arrhythmias, heart block Dose-related nystagmus, diplopia, lethargy, folic acid deficiency, and hyperglycemia Non-dose-related gingival hyperplasia, vitamin D deficiency, peripheral neuropathy, folic acid deficiency, and rash	rash, sedation, dizziness, fatigue, nausea/vomiting, Stevens Johnson Syndrome, hyponatremia, SIADH, diarrhea, diaphoresis	change in menstrual cycle, fatigue, nausea/vomiting, diarrhea, abdominal cramps, anorexia, thrombocytopenia, hepatic failure	dizziness, ataxia, fatigue

Suggested Readings:

Willmore LJ. Post-traumatic epilepsy. In: Evans R, editor. Neurology and Trauma. Philadelphia: W.B. Saunders; 1996.

Annegers JF, Hauser WA, et. al. A population-based study of seizures after traumatic brain injuries. New England Journal of Medicine 1998; 338(1):20-24.

Pohlmann-Eden B, Bruckmeir J. Predictors and dynamics of post-traumatic epilepsy. Acta Neurologica Scandinavia 1997; 95(5):257-262.

Temkin NR, Surreya SD, et. al. A randomized, double-blind study of phenytoin for the prevention of post-traumatic seizures. New England Journal of Medicine 1990; 323(8):497-502.

Hernandez TD, Naritoku DK. Seizures, epilepsy, and functional recovery after traumatic brain injury. Neurology 1997; 48:803-806.

Schierhowt E, et. al. Prophylactic anti-epileptic agents after head injury: a systemic review. Journal of Neurology, Neurosurgery and Psychiatry 1998; 64:108-111.

Jennett B. Epilepsy after non-missile head injuries. 2nd ed. Chicago: William Hieremann; 1975.

Chapter 9

Upper Motor Neuron Syndrome and Spasticity

Mark Kaplan, MD

The upper motor neuron syndrome consists of positive and negative findings. Positive manifestations include spasticity, athetosis, primitive reflexes, rigidity, and dystonia. Negative findings include weakness, paralysis and fatigue.

Spasticity, an abnormality of muscle tone, is common in traumatic brain injury (TBI). It is characterized by a velocity-dependent resistance to passive joint movement. Other clinical findings include hyperactive muscle stretch reflexes and clonus. Many persons with TBI also experience flexor and cutaneo-motor spasms. Although these abnormalities of motor control are not considered manifestations of spasticity, they may respond to many of the same management strategies. In the chronic phase of TBI, an increase in spasticity or spasms may be secondary to medical complications such as urinary tract infections, bowel impaction, or syrinx.

Measuring Spasticity

The Ashworth and Modified Ashworth Scales are the most commonly used scoring instruments and are based on findings during clinical examination. The Spasm Frequency Score is based on the reporting of the individual experiencing abnormalities in muscle tone. Researchers use electrophysiological parameters, such as F-wave and H-reflex measurements (threshold, latency, amplitude, etc.), to quantify spasticity. Changes in electrophysiological measurements, however, may not correlate with clinical or functional improvements. Some studies have also utilized the pendulum test. This test involves placing the examinee in a supine position with the legs hanging over the edge of the plinth. The leg is allowed to fall, and knee movement is assessed with an electrogoniometer.

Modified Ashworth Scale

0 = No increase in muscle tone

1 = Slight increase in muscle tone, manifested as a catch-and-release or by minimal resistance at the end of range of motion

1+ = Slight increase in muscle tone, manifested by catch, followed by minimal resistance throughout the remainder (less than half) of the range of motion

2 = More marked increase in muscle tone throughout most of the range of motion, but the affected part is easily moved

3 = Considerable increase in muscle tone; passive movement difficult

4 = Affected part(s) rigid

Spasm Frequency Score

0 = No spasms

1 = Mild spasm induced by stimulation

2 = Infrequent, full spasm occurring less than once per hour

3 = Spasms occurring more than once per hour

4 = Ten or more spasms per hour, or continuous contraction

Contracture and Spasticity

Many times, contracture and spasticity coexist. Increased muscle tone leads to diminished movement. The result is a cycle that, if untreated, can have deleterious consequences.

Upper Motor Neuron Syndrome and Function

Not all the manifestations of upper motor neuron syndrome require treatment. Sometimes, spasticity and spasms can be beneficial. For example, a patient may use knee extensor spasticity to assist in transferring from a sitting to a standing position. Spasticity of knee extensors may also increase stability during the stance phase of gait. Spasms may be used to assist with bed mobility. Alternatively, increased muscle tone can be deleterious. For example, spasticity may contribute to a poor standing position, which could contribute to contractures and skin breakdown. Flexor spasms of the lower extremity may cause a person with TBI to strike a limb against the leg rests of a wheelchair.

Indications for Treatment of Spasticity

- Decrease pain
- Improve nursing care
- Improve hygiene
- Minimize contractures
- Assist in prevention and healing of pressure ulcers
- Improve seating
- Improve gait and transfers
- Improve self-care activities

Areas of Skin Breakdown Associated With Spasticity

Muscle Group	Area of Potential Skin Breakdown
Shoulder adductors	Axilla
Elbow flexors	Antecubital fossa
Finger flexors	Palm
Hip adductors	Perineum
Knee flexors	Sacrum, heels

Pain and Spasticity

Spasticity may produce pain directly or due to the prolonged contraction of a muscle. Contractures and pressure ulcers can cause pain, which may increase nociceptive afferent impulses and lead to further spasticity.

Treating Spasticity

The treatments for spasticity include physical, medical and surgical interventions. The first step in treating spasticity is to recognize and manage stimuli that may be contributing to increased tone, including urinary tract infections, bladder stones, fecal impaction, heterotopic ossification, or pressure ulcers.

Positioning

Tone may be affected by head and body positions. The tonic neck and vestibular reflexes may be useful in modulating spasticity. For example, some persons with TBI have diminished tone in the partially recumbent position. As such, this position is incorporated into wheelchair-sitting strategies. Casting or splinting an extremity may also diminish spasticity.

Modalities

Cryotherapy and electrical stimulation can reduce spasticity for several hours after application. Sustained cold (i.e., 20 minutes) over a muscle group may decrease spasticity. Alternatively, quick cooling and electrical stimulation of an antagonist of a spastic muscle group may result in reciprocal inhibition and thereby decrease muscle tone. Many individuals with TBI cannot communicate effectively due to cognitive impairment. Therefore, in order to prevent injury, modalities must be prescribed with extreme caution.

Stretching

A stretching program can minimize tone. It should be incorporated into the individual's daily routine. When stretching muscles, a terminal sustained stretch is essential for diminishing tone. The benefit of stretching may last throughout the day.

Medications

The benefits of medications must be balanced against potential cognitive and non-cognitive side effects (Table 1). The annual cost of therapy (i.e., medications, required laboratory tests, repeat physician visits, etc.) must be considered in treatment decisions.

Most clinicians would recommend dantrolene sodium (Dantrium) or tizanidine (Zanaflex) as the first-line agent. The mechanism of action of dantrolene sodium is to diminish calcium release at the level of the sarcoplasmic recticulum. Alternatively, tizanidine, a new agent, is thought to act as an alpha-2 adrenergic agonist. In addition, when compared to tizanidine, dantrolene sodium is more likely to be associated with muscle weakness. Dantrolene sodium also has the potential to cause significant liver toxicity, thus liver function tests should be monitored. Treatment with tizanidine may result in sedation and/or somnolence and may increase serum levels of phenytoin. Furthermore, tizanidine should be used with caution in patients on antihypertensive medications.

Benzodiazepines, such as diazepam, are associated with diminished attention and memory. In addition, long-term benzodiazepines may be associated with dependence. As such, benzodiazepines must be used cautiously in people with TBI.

Baclofen is not a suitable medication in TBI; however, this agent is appropriate for spasticity related to pathology in the spinal cord.

Table 1
Anti-Spasticity Medications

Medication	tizanidine	clonidine	dantrolene sodium	diazepam	baclofen
Brand Name	Zanaflex	Catapres (oral) Catapres TTS (weekly patch)	Dantrium	Valium	Lioresal
Mechanism of Action	alpha-2 agonist (centrally acting)	alpha-2 agonist (centrally acting)	Inhibits Ca2+ release	GABA facilitation	GABA analogue
Starting Dose	2 mg bid	0.1 mg PO bid 0.1 mg/24-hour patch	25 mg qd	2.5 mg bid	2.5 mg bid
Maximum Dose*	36 mg/day	2.4 mg/day 0.3 mg/24-hour patch	400 mg/day	60 mg/day	80 mg/day
Montly Cost Range** **Brand name**	$15.47 – $245.46	$39.79 – $285.48 $26.28 – $80.73	$25.74 – $172.48	$12.94 – $270.89	$11.58– $128.63
Generic	no generic	$12.98 – $91.70 no generic patch	no generic	$4.45 – $41.64	$7.79 – $70.79
Common Side Effects	drowsiness weakness dry mouth mild hypotension	weakness sedation constipation skin rash dry mouth pruritus orthostatic hypotension withdrawal hypertension	weakness sedation dizziness parasthesia nausea diarrhea hepatitis	sedation weakness depression ataxia memory loss dependence	sedation fatigue weakness nausea dizziness parasthesia decreased seizure threshold hallucinations and seizures if withdrawn abruptly

Table adapted from Whyte J, Robinson KM. Pharmacologic management. In: Glenn MB, Hyte J, editors. The practical management of spasticity in children and adults. Malvern, PA: Lea and Febinger; 1990: 222.

*Manfacturers' recommended maximum dose. Some clinicians prescribe higher doses.

**Ranging from initial to maximum dose. Source: Boston Medical Center Outpatient Pharmacy.

Nerve Blocks

Nerve blocks involve injecting a medication close to a nerve to cause temporary or permanent dysfunction. A temporary nerve block can be completed with lidocaine and bupivacaine. This may allow a clinician to evaluate the potential benefits of a nerve block and facilitate the use of other interventions such as serial casting or dynamic splinting. To perform a longer acting nerve block (chemical neurolysis), agents such as phenol and ethanol can be employed.

Nerve blocks can be performed at any anatomically accessible nerve. It is possible to block nerve fibers at the root, plexus or peripheral nerve. Some muscle groups (e.g., iliopsoas) cannot be practically blocked at a distal site, so the neurolysis must be completed at the nerve root (Figure 9.1).

Nerve blocks completed on sensorimotor nerves can result in unwanted dysesthesia and, rarely, anesthesia. Reducing sensory input, however, may be beneficial, as nociceptive inputs sometimes exacerbate spasticity. A motor branch block is a type of chemical neurolysis in which the most distal motor branches of a peripheral nerve are blocked. Motor branch blocks require more needle insertions and can be tedious to perform. There is, however, a lower risk of sensory complications. Other complications from nerve blocks include weakness and sensitivity to the injected agent. Phenol blocks can lead to fibrosis of the nerve and make future nerve blocks at the same site more difficult.

Paravertebral nerve root blocks have more potential side effects. If, during a lumbar paravertebral block, the subarachnoid space is inadvertently compromised, incontinence, sexual dysfunction, and ascending paralysis are possible.

The duration of effect from chemical neurolysis is variable. On average, the effects of the procedure should last between three and nine months. In some individuals, however, the benefits persist for many years. Nerve blocks should be used as part of a comprehensive rehabilitation treatment program; by adding a stretching program, the benefits may be prolonged.

Localization of the nerve is critical for a successful nerve block. The closer the medication is delivered to the nerve, the less medication is required and fewer side effects are likely. The site of injection can be localized with a variable intensity pulse stimulator. A needle coated with teflon (except at the tip) is attached to a syringe. Current is delivered through the needle by a stimulator. As the needle approaches the nerve, a muscle contraction will be elicited. The closer the needle is to the nerve, the less current will be required. With this technique, the medication can be delivered very close to the nerve.

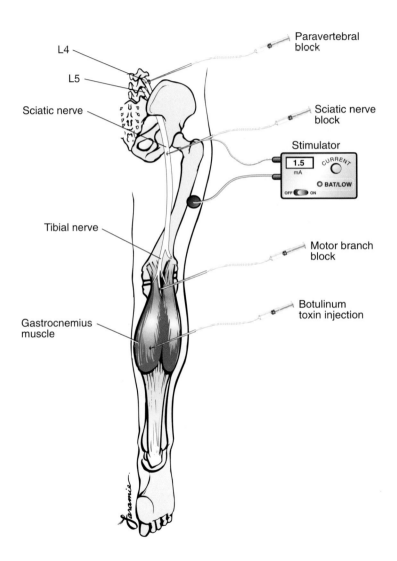

Figure 9.1
Nerve Block

Paravertebral block

L4

L5

Sciatic nerve block

Sciatic nerve

Stimulator

1.5
mA

CURRENT

BAT/LOW

OFF   ON

Tibial nerve

Motor branch block

Botulinum toxin injection

Gastrocnemius muscle

Nerve blocks are commonly performed on muscles innervated by the median, ulnar, obturator, sciatic and tibial nerves. In general, blocking a motor branch is preferred to a mixed sensorimotor nerve.

Botulinum Toxin

The Clostridium botulinum bacterium produces a neurotoxin. When pharmacological preparations of this agent are injected into muscle fibers, there is inhibition of the release of acetylcholine. The result is a neuromuscular blockade with a subsequent decrease in muscle strength and tone.

There are seven serotypes that are antigenically distinct. Currently, botulinum serotype A is commercially available. This preparation requires storage in a freezer and must be reconstituted with normal saline. A botulinum serotype B preparation, which is currently under review by the FDA, will be supplied in a manner that does not require reconstitution. It is generally stored in the refrigerator; however, it is also stable for six months at room temperature.

Botulinum injection treatment, unlike a nerve block, does not require the use of a stimulator. Some clinicians, however, use EMG signals to assist in muscle localization. Risks of injection include reaction to the injectant, bleeding, and infection. This procedure has a duration of effect from one to six months and may be more appropriate for patients soon after injury. The onset of effect typically occurs several days after injection, and the maximum effect is obtained over a period of several weeks. This may be of benefit in allowing patients to gradually adapt to their new muscle strength. Disadvantages include the high cost relative to anesthetic or phenol injection. Subsequent injections may become less effective due to antibody mediated resistance to the botulinum toxin.

Baclofen Pump

Intrathecal baclofen delivery may be effective in patients whose spasticity is not controlled by other means. A temporary catheter is placed into the intrathecal space and a 50 microgram test dose of baclofen is given. A 100 microgram dose can be tried if the lower dose is ineffective and there are no significant side effects. If effective, a permanent catheter is implanted. The pump, with a reservoir, is placed subcutaneously and refilled at one- to three-month intervals. Potential side effects include infection, catheter breakage, drowsiness, hypotension, and weakness. With an overdose, respiratory depression is possible.

Surgical Treatment

Destructive neurosurgical procedures, such as rhizotomy or cordotomy, are rarely performed. Orthopedic procedures can be considered in selected cases. Irreversible procedures should not be performed until neurological recovery has plateaued, typically up to one year post-injury.

Suggested Readings:

Bohannon RW, Smith MB. Interrater reliability of a Modified Ashworth Scale of muscle spasticity. Physical Therapy 1987; 67:206-207.

Kaplan M. Tizanidine: another tool in the management of spasticity. Journal of Head Trauma Rehabilitation 1997; 12(5):93-97.

Glenn MB, Hyte J, editors. The practical management of spasticity in children and adults. Malvern, PA: Lea and Febinger; 1990.

Meyethaler JM, Guin-Renfroe S, Grabb P, Hadley MN. Long-term continuously infused intrathecal baclofen for spastic-dystonic hypertonia in traumatic brain injury: 1-year experience. Archives of Physical Medicine & Rehabilitation 1999 Jan; 80(1):13-9.

Palmer DT, Horn LJ, Harmon RL. Botulinum toxin treatment of lumbrical spasticity: a brief report. American Journal of Physical Medicine & Rehabilitation 1998 Jul-Aug; 77(4):348-50.

Dall JT, Harmon RL, Quinn CM. Use of clonidine for treatment of spasticity arising from various forms of brain injury: a case series. Brain Injury 1996 Jun; 10(6):453-8.

Hill J. The effects of casting on upper extremity motor disorders after brain injury. American Journal of Occupational Therapy 1994 Mar; 48(3):219-24.

Price R, Lehmann JF, Boswell-Bessette S, Burleigh A, deLauteur BJ. Influence of cryotherapy on spasticity at the human ankle. Archives of Physical Medicine & Rehabilitation 1993 Mar; 74(3):300-4.

Pinder RM, Brodgen RN, Speight TM, Avery GS. Dantrolene sodium: a review of its pharmacological properties and therapeutic efficacy in spasticity. [Review] Drugs 1997 Jan; 13(1):3-23.

Chapter 10

Heterotopic Ossification

Douglas E. Garland, MD
Emilia Semenov, MD

The term neurogenic heterotopic ossification (HO) is preferred to such terms as ectopic ossification, paraosteoarthropathy, or myositis ossificans when discussing the formation of new bone near joints as a consequence of traumatic brain injury (TBI). Heterotopic refers to the occurrence of this bone formation in more than one area.

Pathogenesis

Although the pathogenesis of HO is not clearly understood, it involves the metaplasia of mesenchymal cells into osteoblasts. Microscopically, the bone is a true "ossific" process, progressing de novo to new bone formation rather than to calcification of soft tissue. This condition can be present in a number of conditions in addition to TBI, including spinal cord injury, hemorrhagic stroke, and burns. Local trauma to muscle and joints and fractures of bones can also precipitate HO. In TBI, the presence of concomitant fractures, significant soft tissue injury, and spasticity increase the likelihood of developing HO.

The genetic predisposition of HO formation is supported by research into the hereditary disorder fibrodysplasia ossificans progressiva (FOP). This condition is inherited as an autosomal dominant trait with full penetrance and variable expression. It is a disorder of connective tissue, with skeletal malformations and HO. The natural history of HO associated with FOP has similarities to the natural history of HO from other causes, especially neurogenic HO.

The association of human leukocyte antigens (HLA) with neurogenic HO has been documented. An increased prevalence of HLA-B18 and HLA-B27 antigens has been reported in some patients with HO. Follow-up studies, however, have not confirmed these findings.

Clinical Presentation

The reported incidence of HO in TBI varies greatly depending on the hospital or medical center, severity of injury, and method of detection (i.e., clinical examination vs. bone scan). Clinically significant HO that causes substantial limitation of joint range affects approximately 10 percent to 20 percent of people with TBI. Some studies report a 76 percent incidence in patients with severe TBI. Ankylosis is rare (perhaps occurring in less than 10 percent of all HO lesions). Although there are exceptions, HO is diagnosed within six months of the TBI.

HO usually presents in the paralyzed or spastic extremities. Clinical findings include erythema, pain and swelling. Other manifestations include decreased joint range of movement, increased spasticity, and low-grade fevers. HO can cause nerve compression (this is most common with a lesion medial to the elbow compromising the ulnar nerve). The ectopic ossification, when present proximate to bony prominences, may contribute to skin ulcers. Differential diagnoses include deep venous thrombosis, cellulitis, reflex sympathetic dystrophy, abscess, septic joint, hematoma and tumor.

In TBI, the location of HO is equally divided between the upper and lower extremities. HO is often present at fracture sites in TBI. Common locations in the upper extremities include the shoulder and elbow. At the shoulder, the lesion is usually at the inferiomedial aspect. If there is a clavicular fracture or acromioclavicular separation, HO may result in ossification of the coracoclavicular ligament. Forearm fractures are associated with HO formation across the synostosis. Dislocated elbow injuries may result in HO at the medial collateral ligament. In the hip, HO commonly forms inferiomedially, anterolaterally and posteriorly to the joint. Hip dislocations and acetabular fractures are associated with a higher risk of para-articular HO. In TBI, ossific lesions can be present around the knee joint; the lesion at this site is most commonly located medially.

Diagnosis

Elevated levels of serum alkaline phosphatase (SAP) are associated with clinically significant HO. Elevated SAP levels are more common in hip lesions when compared to upper extremity HO. SAP levels begin to rise to the upper limits of normal within the first two weeks of injury. At three weeks, the SAP levels may exceed normal values, and the elevation may persist for up to five months. The SAP level parallels the clinical course of HO.

The three-phase radionuclide bone scan is the best method for early detection and confirmation of HO. This test requires an intravenous injection of 99mTc-labeled methylene diphosphonate. The radioisotope concentrates in areas of increased bone activity. The three phases of a bone scan are the dynamic blood flow phase (nuclear angiogram), immediate static phase (blood pool phase), and the delayed static phase. Abnormalities in the first two phases of the bone scan will present prior to abnormalities in the third phase. Clinicians should insist on a three-phase study, and not a single static phase study. A three-phase bone scan can detect HO as early as two to three weeks after the onset of the lesion.

Radiographs may provide confirmatory evidence of HO. Although plain films may detect HO as early as three weeks after injury, radiographic detection may not be confirmatory until two months after the initial clinical presentation.

The precise role of computed tomography (CT) scanning as a clinical tool for diagnosis and a measure of maturation of HO is not established. CT scanning clearly defines HO and its relationship to muscle, vessels and nerves. This study should be considered prior to surgical excision.

Treatment

The clinical significance of HO varies from patient to patient, and management decisions must be individualized. In some individuals, the HO is of little functional significance and requires no intervention. Others suffer from multiple lesions that significantly impair function. The majority of patients can be satisfactorily managed with physical therapy and medications.

Physical Interventions

Physical therapy can be helpful in the management of HO. The goal is to maintain functional range of movement. The affected joints should be gently moved through functional range. On occasion, the amount of spasticity is so severe that joint range of movement can only be achieved under anesthesia.

Medical Management

Prophylactic HO treatment with medications for every TBI is probably not warranted. If there is a clinical suspicion of HO, then a bone scan is appropriate.

Patients diagnosed with HO can be treated with etidronate disodium (EHDP). This medication is a structural analog of inorganic phosphate and limits ossification by blocking the formation of hydroxyapatite crystals. The oral dose is 20 mg/kg per day and may be given in one dose or in two divided doses for a period of up to six months. Some clinicians recommend that initial treatment be with intravenous EHDP (300 mg per day) for the first three days, followed by oral therapy. The most common side effects of EHDP are nausea, vomiting, diarrhea and abdominal discomfort. Treatment with EHDP can contribute to osteoporosis and impair fracture healing. In studies with dogs, pathologic fractures have developed after nine months of treatment.

Nonsteroidal anti-inflammatory drugs (NSAID) have not been proven to decrease the incidence of HO associated with TBI. NSAID may be indicated subsequent to surgical resection for a period of three to six months. The optimal dose of NSAID has not been clearly demonstrated. The benefits of NSAID must be balanced against the potential side effects, including possible gastrointestinal hemorrhages. Indomethacin is the preferred NSAID, at 25 mg three times a day. Alternate choices are ibuprofen (300 - 800 mg tid) and aspirin (650 mg tid).

Surgery

Surgery is appropriate in selected cases that are refractory to conservative management. Surgical indications include functionally diminished joint mobility, impaired sitting, profound pain, progressive nerve compromise, and significant spasticity. Surgical treatment may range from a wedge resection to the complete removal of the lesion. The goal is not to eradicate the ectopic bone, but rather to achieve preoperative functional goals.

The timing of surgical intervention in HO associated with TBI is critical. Patients at low Rancho Los Amigos Scale of Cognitive Functioning levels and with significant upper motor neuron syndrome findings are more likely to have recurrence of a lesion after surgical treatment. As such, surgical intervention should be deferred (perhaps up to 18 months) until no further neurological recovery can be reasonably expected.

Postoperative prophylaxis is necessary, especially for patients in prolonged coma with severe abnormalities in tone. Combination therapy with radiation treatment and medications is desirable. Radiation therapy at 600 - 750 rads in single or divided doses is appropriate. As well, EHDP or NSAID are necessary for a period of three to six months.

Suggested Readings:

Garland DE. Clinical observations on fractures and heterotopic ossification in the spinal cord and traumatic brain injury populations. Clinical Orthopedics 1998; 233:86-100.

Garland, DE. A clinical perspective of common forms of acquired heterotopic ossification. Clinical Orthopedics 1991; 263:13-29.

Garland DE, Blum CE, Waters RL. Periatricular heterotopic ossification in head injured adults: incidence and location. Journal of Bone and Joint Surgery 1980; 62A:1153-1146.

Garland DE, Hanscom DA, Keenan MA, Someth C, Moore T. Resection of heterotopic ossification in the adult with head trauma. Journal of Bone and Joint Surgery 1985; 67A:1261-1269.

Garland, DE. Heterotopic ossification in traumatic brain injury. In: Ashley M, Krych D, editors. Traumatic brain injury rehabilitation. Boca Raton, FL: CRC Press; 1995; 119-129.

Jensen LL, Halar E, Little JW, Brooke MM. Special review: neurogenic hetero-topic ossification. American Journal of Physical Medicine 1988; 66(6):351-363.

Kolessar DJ, Katz SD, Keenan MA. Functional outcome following surgical resection of heterotopic ossification in patients with brain injury. Journal of Head Trauma Rehabilitation 1996; 11(4):78-87.

Orzel JA, Rudd TG. Heterotopic bone formation: clinical, laboratory, and imaging correlation. Journal of Nuclear Medicine 1985; 26:125-132.

Sarafis KA, Karatzas GD, Yotis CL. Ankylosed hips caused by heterotopic ossification after traumatic brain injury: a difficult problem. Journal of Trauma 1999; 46(1):104-109.

Spielman G, Gennarelli TA, Rogers CR. Disodium etidronate: its role in pre-venting heterotopic ossification in severe head injury. Archives of Physical Medicine and Rehabilitation 1983; 64:539-542.

Tsur A, Sazbon L, Lotern M. Relationship between muscular tone, movement and periarticular new bone formation in postcoma-unaware (PC-U) patients. Brain Injury 1996; 10(4):259-262.

Chapter 11

Contracture Management

Steven Nussbaum, MD

Pathology

Contractures are defined as a fixed loss of passive joint range of movement secondary to pathology of connective tissue, tendons, ligaments, muscles, joint capsules and cartilage. Traumatic, inflammatory, ischemic or infectious factors can cause collagen proliferation. These collagen fibers may initially be deposited in a disorganized manner. If the joint is taken through full functional range (either actively or passively), the newly-deposited collagen will organize in a linear fashion. Alternatively, if the joint is immobilized, the collagen matrix will organize in a tightly packed manner, and a contracture will result.

Classification

Contractures can be classified as arthrogenic, soft tissue or myogenic. Arthrogenic contractures are caused by pathology involving the intrinsic joint components. Examples include cartilage damage secondary to osteoarthritis, or joint incongruency as the result of an intra-articular fracture. Arthrogenic contractures generally cause range of movement restrictions in multiple directions.

Soft tissue contractures result in the shortening of tendons, ligaments and skin. These contractures generally cause restriction of movement in one direction.

Myogenic contractures can be divided into intrinsic and extrinsic lesions. Intrinsic muscle contractures are secondary to a primary disorder of muscle fibers. An example would be muscular dystrophy in which histologically abnormal muscle is present. Most traumatic brain injury (TBI) patients suffer from extrinsic muscle contractures as a result of muscles being placed in a shortened position for extended periods of time. The muscle, however, is histologically normal. Factors that can lead to extrinsic contractures include spasticity, immobility, improper positioning, and pain. Heterotopic ossification can also cause extrinsic myogenic contractures.

Common Locations of Contractures

In the lower extremities, ankle plantarflexion, hip flexion, and knee flexion contractures are common. In the upper extremities, elbow flexion and supination contractures are possible. Some patients may also develop shoulder adduction and internal rotation contractures. Muscles that cross multiple joints, such as the biceps, hamstrings, tensor fascia lata, and gastrocnemius, are predisposed to contracture formation.

Prevention of Contractures

Contractures can be prevented with early mobilization, range of movement exercises, proper positioning, and orthotic devices. Contracture prevention requires the coordinated effort of the medical, nursing and therapy services. Patients must be encouraged to get out of bed as soon as practical. The therapeutic exercise program must be tailored to the patient's level of injury. If the patient is capable, ambulation with devices should be encouraged. Patient and caregiver education emphasizing the importance of performing a home stretching program is essential.

Splinting is an effective adjunctive treatment for contracture management. It is not, however, a substitute for a comprehensive rehabilitation treatment program. Orthotic devices can be prescribed to maintain positioning of the hands, elbows, knees and ankles. Patient comfort is essential for a successful splinting program. Skin irritation and pain can result in non-compliance. After initial fabrication of the orthosis, the patient should be monitored every 30 minutes for problems with skin tolerance. If pressure areas are not detected, a two-hour wearing schedule is initiated. The patient may increase the wearing schedule to a full night as skin tolerance allows.

Improper bed positioning may contribute to contractures. The supine position encourages hip flexion and ankle plantarflexion contractures. Placing a pillow under a patient's knees will encourage hip and knee flexion contractures. Another bed position to avoid is one that encourages extreme adduction and internal rotation of the shoulder. Proper bed positioning can minimize contracture formation. Patients should be advised to lie prone in bed to minimize hip flexion contractures. When in bed, the shoulder should be placed in abduction and some external rotation. This can be achieved with strategic placement of pillows. The progression of ankle flexion contractures can be prevented with ankle foot orthosis. Flexion and supination contractures at the elbow can be prevented with resting night splints or bivalved casts, both of which promote elbow extension and pronation.

Proper wheelchair seating and positioning are also essential in preventing the formation of contractures. Contractures and subluxation of the shoulder can be prevented with the placement of armrests and lapboards on the wheelchair. Forward placement of the armrest encourages extension of the elbow.

The pelvis should be maintained with a slight anterior tilt, thus encouraging normal lordosis in the lumbar spine and kyphosis in the thoracic spine. A posterior pelvic tilt will encourage kyphosis of the lumbar spine, causing the head and neck to lean forward. Extensions, also called hip blocks, placed on a wheelchair laterally keep the pelvis symmetrical and help to align the lower extremities. A short hip block stabilizes the pelvis while a long hip block prevents excessive abduction. Leg straps can be used to prevent adduction of the lower extremities while sitting in the wheelchair. Footrest height can be adjusted to change the position of the ankle, knee and hip. The trunk can be stabilized by utilizing laterally placed trunk supports and by modifying the seat to recline 10 degrees.

Treatment of Contractures

Every reasonable step should be taken to prevent contractures. Once a contracture has formed, however, a variety of interventions are available. The factors that are contributing to contracture formation, such as pain, spasticity, inflammation and improper positioning, should be treated. Treatments can be divided into three groups: physical, medical and surgical.

Physical interventions include therapeutic heat (i.e., ultrasound) prior to a stretching program. A terminal sustained stretch is essential. Caution must be used with therapeutic heat in areas with impaired sensation. Regional osteoporosis may also have caused fragile bones, and vigorous stretching may lead to a fracture.

Serial casting (Figure 11.1) or dynamic splinting can be an adjunctive therapy to a stretching program. Serial casting utilizes a plaster cast that is applied to a limb that has been pre-stretched. The cast is subsequently removed in three to five days, and a new cast is placed after the limb is stretched another five to 10 degrees. This process continues until the contracture has been reduced. Serial casting should be discontinued if pain or pressure ulcers develop. Dynamic splinting utilizes splints with movable parts to counter contracting forces. Dynasplints and outrigger splints are examples of dynamic splints.

In refractory cases, orthopedic surgical procedures, such as joint manipulation, tendon release, and tendon lengthening, can be considered. If pain or spasticity are contributing to contractures, these conditions should be managed appropriately.

Figure 11.1
Serial Casting

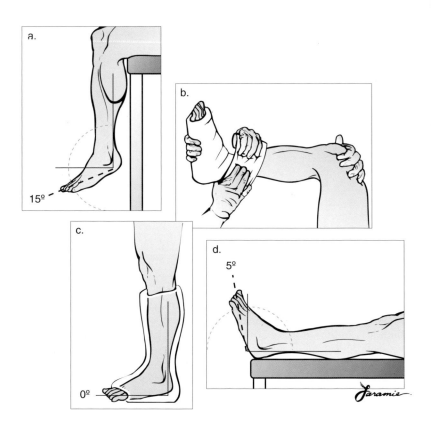

Suggested Readings:

Halar E, Bell K. Contracture and other deleterious effects of immobility. In: DeLisa J, editor: Rehabilitation medicine principles and practice. Philadelphia: Williams & Wilkins; 1988; 448-455.

Halar E. Rehabilitation's relationship to inactivity. In: Kottke F, Lehmann J, editors. Krusen's handbook of physical medicine and rehabilitation. Philadelphia: W.B. Saunders; 1990.

Chapter 12

Impairments of Olfaction and Vision

Kimberly G. Chagnon, MS, ANP

Impairments of olfaction and vision are common in traumatic brain injury (TBI). Although these conditions are often managed in conjunction with other specialists (i.e., otolaryngologists, neurosurgeons, ophthalmologists), it is important for rehabilitation clinicians to have some understanding of the fundamental concepts of smell and vision. Impairments of these two senses are sometimes not clinically appreciated during the acute hospital admission, but become apparent during the rehabilitation course. As severely injured TBI patients are unable to communicate, it is difficult to accurately ascertain an individual's ability to see and smell.

Impairment of Olfaction

The olfactory response originates in specialized chemical receptors located in the mucous membranes of the upper nasal cavity. The olfactory nerve (CN I) contains delicate demyelinated fibers that pass along the cribriform plate and terminate at the olfactory bulb, which is situated in the hippocampal region. Damage to the olfactory pathways impairs both the ability to smell and taste.

When all TBI are considered, the incidence of anosmia (loss of the sense of smell) is estimated to be between 2.5 percent and 10.5 percent. In severe TBI, the incidence is estimated to be up to 30 percent. Although anosmia is more likely with severe TBI, trivial blows to the frontal and occipital areas of the brain can often result in olfactory compromise. Fractures of the cribriform plate, which may be associated with cerebrospinal fluid rhinorrhea, may cause abnormalities of smell. Fifty percent of TBI patients with anosmia will recover during the first three months post-injury. Some patients, however, may never experience total resolution.

Anosmia is often unrecognized because physicians rarely test the sense of smell during a routine physical examination. To assess impairments of smell, obscure one nostril; saturate a cotton ball with peppermint, lemon oil or clove; and ask the patient to identify the odor. Test each nostril separately. Alcohol should not be used because it will stimulate noxious receptors and is, therefore, not a test for olfactory function.

Both damage to the olfactory response and an associated impairment of taste have functional consequences. Anosmia may make dining unpalatable, thus reducing caloric intake. In some patients with frontal lobe injuries, agitation may be precipitated by hunger. Consequently, the rehabilitation team has to manage potentially avoidable behavioral episodes.

Impairments of Vision

The visual system includes the optic nerves, visual pathways, and visual centers of the occipital lobe. The optic nerve (CN II) is part of the peripheral nervous system and is the largest of the cranial nerves. It is injured in approximately 1.6 percent of all head injuries. The optic nerves arise from the photoreceptors in the retina and join the retina at the optic disc or fundus. The visual pathways then continue posterior to a point at which the optic nerves converge. This area of convergence, above the sella turcica of the sphenoid bone, is called the optic chiasm. At the chiasm, a partial departure occurs, with the medial portion of each optic nerve crossing to the other side. The tracts then proceed posterolaterally to terminate in the lateral geniculate bodies.

The visual cortex is located in the calcarine fissure of the occipital lobe and is considered the primary visual area of the brain. The visual cortex is concerned with visual perception, visual fixation, and involuntary eye movements. Even though the occipital lobe is the predominant visual center, other areas of the brain are involved with visual cognition. The frontal lobe influences eye movements. The parietal lobe is involved in processing visual-spatial information. The peristriate region of the temporal lobe is involved with visual impressions and memories.

Although relatively minor trauma can cause injury to the optic nerve, most optic nerve injuries are associated with severe TBI. In civilian life, penetrating injuries and blunt wounds account for approximately 25 percent and 75 percent of optic nerve injuries, respectively. Many times, the trajectory of a missile spares the cortex, yet it damages one or more cranial nerves.

Not all TBI visual impairments are related to neurological pathology. Other causes include traumatic lens dislocation, ruptured globe, corneal abrasions, and anterior chamber hemorrhage (hyphema).

Typical complaints associated with CN II compromise include monocular blindness, visual field deficits, diminished visual acuity, and blurred vision. Impairment of vision can occur immediately after an injury, or it can become apparent several hours to days post-TBI. Many times, patients who have CN II compromise also suffer from CN III, IV or VI pathology. As a result, diplopia is also possible.

Blows that cause occipital lobe injury can cause blindness. Some individuals with injuries to the visual association areas of the brain may develop visual anosognosia (Anton's Syndrome). Affected patients will characteristically deny any visual impairment even though they obviously cannot see.

Suggested Readings:

Keane JR, Baloh RW. Post-traumatic cranial nerve neuropathies. In: Evans RW. Neurology and trauma. Philadelphia, PA: W. B. Saunders; 1996.

Greenberg MS. Handbook of neurosurgery. 4th ed. Lakeland, FL: Greenberg Graphics; 1997.

Narayan RK, Wilberger JE, Povlishock JT, editors. Neurotrauma. New York: McGraw-Hill; 1996.

Chapter 13

Community Reintegration

Troy Scherer

The ultimate goal of a TBI rehabilitation program is to return the individual to his premorbid functional status. Ulitmately, successful return to the community for TBI patients is dependent on several factors, including the ability to perform functional tasks, presence of behavioral and/or cognitive dysfunction, level of family support, and amount of financial resources. TBI patients who are discharged from an acute medical and rehabilitation hospital will usually require continuing rehabilitation services.

Home Discharge

Discharging the patient home is an important programmatic goal. TBI patients are able to return home if there is an adequate amount of supervision and structure. For example, some patients require 24-hour supervision for safety. This is very difficult for some families to provide, but it may be accomplished through coordinated efforts of family and designated (paid or unpaid) caregivers. Physical, occupational and speech-language therapy services can also be provided in the home. In many instances, however, due to the patient's cognitive or behavioral impairments, this arrangement is unsafe or ineffective in providing continuous, structured learning opportunities. Thus, some families may require supportive counseling to understand the need for an alternative discharge (e.g., to a residential care facility, skilled nursing home, etc.).

Outpatient Rehabilitation Clinics

Outpatient rehabilitation clinics provide the least supervised and structured setting outside the home for patients to continue their rehabilitation. Patients who are able to attend scheduled appointments with individual therapists in an outpatient clinic usually have milder functional and behavioral impairments, or have initially sustained only a mild TBI.

Residential Care

TBI patients who require minimal supervision, but need emotional supports and continued structure in their day, may be able to reside in a residential care facility. In this setting, TBI patients live together and assist one another with many daily activities, with the support of a few counselors. Some structured routine is provided, including meal times, assigned chores, group shopping, and recreational outings. Frequently, counselors in some facilities sleep overnight to ensure availability of continuous guidance and support to residents.

Day Treatment Centers

Day treatment centers usually are facilities in which TBI patients are able to spend up to eight hours in a structured, supervised setting with individual and group therapy sessions. At the end of the treatment day, patients return to their homes for the evening to be with family or other care providers. One advantage of day treatment programs is that they allow the TBI patient's treatment team an opportunity to expose the patient to increasingly difficult, but practical, problems in their therapy. For example, patients can practice safety skills in navigating streets or shopping in actual grocery stores. Vocational counseling and rehabilitation are also offered by some day treatment centers.

Skilled Nursing Facilities

As the name suggests, skilled nursing facilities provide 24-hour skilled nursing care. Patients who require this level of supervision and structure are incapable of providing for their own basic needs in a safe or consistent manner. The level of therapies available and staff expertise with TBI vary greatly among different facilities. While there are a few skilled nursing facilities that can provide behavioral programs and cognitive rehabilitation, the majority do not. In addition, the majority of skilled nursing facilities are more suited to geriatric patients than the usually much younger TBI patient. Thus, every effort to identify and transfer TBI patients to an appropriate skilled nursing facility must be made. This may be done in several ways. The local chapter of the National Brain Injury Association will likely be able to identify more appropriate nursing home facilities for TBI patients, if they are available. Regardless of recommendations, families and friends of TBI patients should be encouraged to tour prospective skilled nursing facilities prior to transferring from the acute inpatient TBI program.

Community Support

Community organizations, such as local chapters of the National Brain Injury Association, are recognized as the leading community advocates for persons who have sustained TBI. They provide information regarding clinical and support services in the community.

Financial Support

Private financial support for persons who have sustained TBI is usually limited. Most of this support is from disability insurance benefits, as well as some retirement plans. Some persons may qualify for governmental support in the form of Social Security Disability Insurance (SSDI) or Supplemental Social Security Benefits (SSI). Persons who qualify for SSDI have contributed to the federal Social Security program for five of the last 10 years and are unable to work due to their physical or mental impairments. In contrast, SSI disability benefits are available to all legal residents of the U.S., including those who have not contributed to the Social Security program. SSI is available for persons of limited income and assets.

Medical Benefits

Medical benefits are most often secured through private insurance, Medicaid and Medicare. Private insurance is normally related to employment status at the time the TBI patient was injured. Medicaid is a state-administered program that is partially supported by the federal government. The amount of services available through Medicaid varies greatly from state to state. For example, Massachusetts provides relatively broad coverage, including durable medical equipment (e.g., shower chairs, wheelchairs, etc.) and consumable medical supplies. In some states, Medicaid benefits are more limited, thus creating an economic barrier to returning to the community.

Medicare is administered and funded by the federal government. It is primarily focused on providing care for the elderly (over age 65); however, persons who are disabled and unable to work permanently or for prolonged periods of time could be eligible. It consists of part A and part B. Part A pays for inpatient hospital care, skilled nursing home services, hospice care, and home health services. Part B covers inpatient and outpatient practitioner charges and outpatient diagnostic services. In general, persons who receive SSDI benefits are eligible for Medicare benefits after a two-year waiting period.

Conclusion

In an ideal situation, TBI care is provided in a seamless fashion from acute injury to community reintegration. If the TBI patient's discharge does not provide for this continuity of care, there is a risk for regression of the patient's functional and behavioral skills. As such, a thoughtful clinician must be able to assess a rehabilitation patient's needs in the context of available community resources.

Suggested Readings:

Dixon T. Systems of care for the head injured. In: Horn L, Cope N. Traumatic brain injury, physical medicine and rehabilitation: state of the art reviews (vol. 3, no. 1). Philadelphia: Hanley & Belfus, Inc.; 1989.

Malkmus D, Booth B, Kodimer C. Rehabilitation of the head injured adult: comprehensive cognitive management. Downey, CA: Professional Staff Association of Rancho Los Amigos Hospital, Inc.; 1980.

Livingston M, Brooks N. The burden on families of the brain injured: a review. Journal of Head Trauma 1988; 3(4):6-15.

Chapter 14

Mild Traumatic Brain Injury

Buck H. Woo, PhD

As discussed in chapter 1, mild traumatic brain injury (MTBI) occurs with greater frequency than either moderate or severe TBI. MTBI is a controversial diagnosis, and some physicians are reluctant to acknowledge the presence of this clinical entity. Although its pathophysiological mechanism is unclear, thoughtful practitioners must recognize that the clinical manifestations of MTBI often are unrecognized.

Diagnosis

As with many conditions treated by rehabilitation clinicians, there is controversy in the exact diagnostic criteria for MTBI. The Mild Traumatic Brain Injury Committee of the Head Injury Interdisciplinary Special Interest Group of the American Congress of Rehabilitation Medicine has provided the following criteria (based on the presence of at least one of the following) for the diagnosis of MTBI:

- brief loss of consciousness (less than five minutes) at the time of the accident
- loss of memory before or after the injury
- alteration of mental state at the time of injury (e.g., feeling dazed, disoriented or confused)
- focal neurological deficit(s), which may or may not be transient.

In addition, MTBI can be diagnosed when the severity of the injury does not exceed the following:

- loss of consciousness of approximately 30 minutes or less
- an initial Glasgow Coma Scale score of 13 -15 after 30 minutes
- post-traumatic amnesia not greater than 24 hours.

Symptoms of MTBI may be transient, or they can produce chronic disabilities in a person's social and work lives. Symptoms generally fall into one of three categories: physical symptoms, cognitive deficits, or behavioral and emotional changes. Physical symptoms of MTBI include nausea, vomiting, dizziness, headache, blurred vision, sleep disturbance, poor endurance, and lethargy. Cognitive deficits associated with MTBI are in attention, concentration, perception, memory, language, and executive functions. Finally, behavioral and emotional changes include alterations in emotional lability, disinhibition, irritability, and anger control.

Accurately determining a patient's level of impairment may be difficult. A careful history of the patient's premorbid level of cognitive and emotional functioning from family members and associates is important to determine the diagnostic significance of the patient's presenting behaviors. For example, it is unlikely that a highly labile, disinhibited, and impulsive patient who worked many years as a librarian is functioning at his normal baseline. A neuropsychological evaluation to determine the pattern and magnitude of cognitive and personality changes is recommended to assist in the diagnostic and eventual rehabilitation process.

Treatment of MTBI

In general, MTBI patients benefit from the same principles that guide the treatment of moderate to severe TBI. The treatment of MTBI involves cognitive rehabilitation, neuropharmacology, and counseling. Cognitive rehabilitation should be based on a thorough neuropsychological evaluation in order to understand the patient's pattern of strengths and weaknesses. For example, patients who have visual-organization deficits and intact verbal memory and language skills can be taught to utilize street signs to avoid getting lost in the community.

Neuropharmacologic interventions may be helpful. The use of neurostimulants with low side-effect profiles, such as methylphenidate and amantadine, can be utilized to improve attention and memory. Mood disorders, such as anxiety and depression, often accompany MTBI and will generally respond well to mood stabilizing medications, including valproic acid and antidepressant medications such as sertraline. Please see chapter 7 for more detailed information on neuropharmacology after TBI.

Finally, studies show that many MTBI patients have demonstrated relief of mood disorders and better adjustment in the community when provided with psychotherapeutic interventions, including individual, family and group psychotherapy.

Typically, people with MTBI have an unremarkable standard neurological exam (cranial nerves, reflexes, power, etc.) and normal neuroimaging. As such, some physicians conclude that the patients' symptoms are in the psychiatric sphere of medical practice. In reality, people with MTBI are truly suffering and should receive the appropriate attention of health-care professionals.

Suggested Readings:

Ashley M, Krych D. Traumatic brain injury. Boca Raton, FL: CRC Press; 1995.

Barth J, Macciocchi S, issue editors. Mild traumatic brain injuries. Journal of Head Injury Rehabilitation 1993 Sep; volume 8, number 3.

Chapter 15

Pediatric Traumatic Brain Injury

Steven Williams, MD
Michael Stillman

Introduction

It is axiomatic that children are not "little adults." As such, the management of pediatric traumatic brain injury (TBI) requires a thorough understanding of child development, as well as the clinical and pathophysiological manifestations of a brain injury. Pediatric TBI is a disease that stands at the intersection of rehabilitation medicine, child psychiatry, and general pediatrics. For optimal outcomes, the treatment team must include a variety of disciplines with expertise in pediatric TBI.

Epidemiology

Each year in the United States, approximately 200,000 children require hospitalization due to TBI and nearly 5,000 die as a result of head trauma. The incidence of TBI is lowest in children under the age of five and highest in adolescents. Boys sustain brain injuries twice as often as girls. The major causes of pediatric TBI include falls, motor vehicle collisions, child abuse, and interpersonal violence. Motor vehicle collisions cause a disproportionate rate of TBI-related fatalities.

In general, children with TBI are more likely to be members of dysfunctional families. There is an association between poor parenting and supervision and an increased risk of pediatric TBI. Pediatric TBI may place great financial and emotional burdens on families, which may be compounded in dysfunctional families.

Pathophysiology of Injury

The pathophysiology and surgical management of TBI are described in chapters 2 and 3. As in adults, pediatric TBI can be divided into focal injuries (e.g., frontal contusion, subdural hemorrhage) and diffuse injuries (diffuse axonal injury). In children, however, the disruption of the myelin sheath associated with DAI may be reversible. When compared to adults, children are more prone to developing diffuse cerebral edema and elevated intracranial pressure. Thus, physicians should be particularly vigilant in the clinical assessment and monitoring of children with TBI.

Children suffer from many of the same complications as adults with TBI: post-traumatic seizures, cranial nerve injuries, basal skull fractures, cognitive impairments, and language dysfunction. Unlike adults, however, children are in the process of "growing up." As such, the static and developmental impacts of a particular impairment must be addressed. For example, a three-year-old who suffers from a frontal contusion may have impairment of attention and anger control. As a result, the child may not successfully interact with others on the playground or he may be disruptive in school.

Developmental Issues

An orderly and relatively predictable acquisition and refinement of physical, cognitive and social skills characterize normal child development (Table 1). As the central nervous system matures, children are able to undertake more complex behaviors.

Developmental skills are attained in an age-specific sequential manner; however, there is a normal range of variation among children. To evaluate impairments in children with TBI, the clinician must understand normal childhood development. Children who have experienced TBI may be delayed in attaining developmental milestones, or they may regress.

Motor skills are attained in a cephalocaudal progression. The normal sequence is head control, which is followed by voluntary reaching and grasping. With advancing age, sitting and walking are achieved. Behavior patterns are evolved from generalized movements and responses to more discrete, refined and complex actions.

Four areas of function that are evaluated in developmental assessments include:

- gross motor behavior (i.e., head control, rolling, crawling and walking)
- fine motor-adaptive behavior (i.e., prehension, manipulatory skills such as using a spoon, and utilization of the sensorimotor system in encounters of daily living such as stacking blocks of a similar color)
- language behavior (i.e., vocalization, comprehension and expression)
- personal social behavior (i.e., acquisition of culture-specific appropriate social interaction such as table manners and interacting with other children and adults).

Cognitive and Intellectual Impairments

TBI can result in cognitive and intellectual impairments in children. The more severe the TBI, the more likely that a child will have deficits. Younger patients, given the same type of injury, are more likely to suffer intellectual impairments. For example, children under 10 with severe TBI show significantly lower performance on IQ testing than older children with similar TBI severity. Children with TBI may have deficits in registration, as well as immediate, long-term and remote memory. In addition, some patients may have visual-spatial and visual-motor impairments, as well as diminished hand/eye coordination.

Pediatric TBI can result in a spectrum of communication disorders (e.g., aphasia, dysarthria and impairments in reading and writing). The most common language disorder in pediatric TBI is expressive aphasia. The overwhelming majority of pediatric TBI patients will recover functional language skills, but 25 percent will have some communication deficit.

Post-traumatic behavior changes can be divided into three stages:

1) Early stage behavioral sequelae include agitation and impaired information processing. Patients may exhibit non-purposeful motor activity and verbal outcries. These behaviors are not responsive to sedation. Children with acute TBI may also develop "sleeping beauty syndrome," marked by motionlessness, apathy and unresponsiveness.

2) Middle stage sequelae include intolerance to external stimuli (e.g., "acting out" in response to a loud television), which leads to decreased compliance to instructions from caregivers and increased demands on staff and family.

3) Final stage sequelae result from the patient's awareness of his cognitive impairments. The resulting loss of self-esteem may manifest as depression, anger and risk-taking behaviors.

Conclusion

There are several important issues to be aware of in pediatric TBI, including post-traumatic medical issues, impairment of normal childhood development, and impairments in intellectual and other cognitive functions, which will affect the child for the remainder of his life. These are all major obstacles to be dealt with by the pediatric TBI patient's rehabilitation team and family.

Suggested Readings:

Molnar GE, editor. Pediatric rehabilitation. 2nd ed. Philadelphia: Williams & Wilkins; 1992.

Gennarelli TA. Mechanisms and pathophysiology of cerebral concussion. Journal of Head Trauma Rehabilitation 1986; 2:23-29.

DeLisa JA, Gans BM, Currie DM, Gerber LH, Leonard JA, McPhee WC, Pease WS, editors. Rehabilitation medicine: principles and practice. 2nd ed. Philadelphia: J.B. Lippincott Co.; 1993.

Rosenthal M, Griffith ER, Bond MR, Miller JD, editors. Rehabilitation of adult and child with traumatic brain injury. 2nd ed. Philadelphia: F. A. Davis Co.; 1990.

Wiercisiewski DR, McDeavitt JT. Pulmonary complications of TBI. Journal of Head Trauma Rehabilitation 1998; 13(1):28-35.

Jacob G, Ritz A, Emrich R. Cranial nerve damage after pediatric head trauma: a long term follow-up study of 741 cases. Acta Pediatr Hung 1986; 27:173-187.

Ewing-Cobbs L. Longitudinal neurophsychological outcome in infants and preschoolers with traumatic brain injury. Journal of the International Neuropsychology Society 1997 Nov; 3(36):555-567.

Speech/Language	Cognitive	Emotional

Three-word sentences are usual
Uses future tense
Asks "what," "who," "where"
Follows prepositional commands,
  i.e., "put it under"
Gives full name
May stutter in eagerness
Identifies self as boy or girl
Recognizes three colors
	Preoperational period continues
	Child is capable of:
	— deferred imitation
	— drawing of graphic images
	— mental images
	— verbal evocation of events
	— symbolic play
		Stage of initiative vs. guilt (3-6 yr)
		Deals with issue of genital
		  sexuality

Gives connected account of recent experiences Questions "why," "when," "how" Uses past tense, adjectives, adverbs Knows opposite analogies Repeats four digits		

Fluent speech
Misarticulations of some sounds
  may persist
Gives name, address, age
Defines concrete nouns, by
  composition, classification or use
Follows three-part commands
Has number concepts to 10
		Stage of industry vs. inferiority
		  (5yr-adolescence)
		Adjusts himself to the inorganic
		  laws of the tool world

Shows mastery of grammar Uses proper articulation		Stage of industry vs. inferiority continues

	Period of concrete operational
	  thought (7 yr –adolescence)
	Child is capable of logical
	  thinking	

from Williams & Wilkins.

Age	Gross Motor	Fine Motor-Adaptive	Personal

Newborn	Flexor tone predominates
	In prone, turns head to side
	Automatic reflex walking
	Rounded spine when held sitting
		Hands fisted
		Grasp reflex
		State dependent ability to fix
		  and follow bright object
			Habituation and
			  of state

4 months	Head midline Head held when pulled to sit In prone, lifts head to 90° and lifts chest slightly Turns to supine	Hands mostly open Midline hand play Crude palmar grasp	Recognizes bottle

7 months	Maintains sitting, may lean on arms
	Rolls to prone
	Bears all weight; bounces when
	  held erect
	Cervical lordosis
	Reaches with arm in prone
		Intermediate grasp
		Transfers cube from hand to hand
		Bangs objects
			Differentiates be
			  person and stra
			Holds bottle
			Looks for droppe
			"Talks" to his mi

10 months	Creeps on all fours
	Pivots in sitting
	Stands momentarily
	Slight bow leg
	Cruises
	Increased lumbar lordosis; acute
	  lumbo-sacral angulation
		Pincer grasp, mature thumb to
		  index grasp
		Bangs two cubes held in hands
			Plays peek-a-boo
			Finger feeds
			Chews with rota

14 months	Walks alone, arms in high
	  guard or midguard
	Wide base, excessive knee and
	  hip flexion
	Foot contact on entire sole
	Slight valgus knees and feet
	Pelvic tilt and rotation
		Piles two cubes
		Scribbles spontaneously
		Holds crayon full length in palm
		Casts objects
			Uses spoon with
			  and spilling
			Removes a garm

18 months	Arms at low guard
	Mature supporting base and heal
	  strike
	Seats self in chair
	Walks backwards
		Emerging hand dominance
		Crude release
		Holds crayon butt end in palm
		Dumps raisin from bottle
		  spontaneously
			Imitates housew
			Carries, hugs do
			Drinks from cup

2 yr	Begins running Walks up and down stairs alone Jumps on both feet in place	Hand dominance is usual Builds eight-cube tower Aligns cubes horizontally Imitates vertical line Places pencil shaft between thumb and fingers Draws with arm and wrist action	Pulls on garmen Uses spoon well Opens door turn Feeds doll with b Toilet training u

Table 1
n Child Development

Social	Speech/Language	Cognitive	Emotional
...ome control	Cry State dependent quieting and head turning to rattle or voice	Sensorimotor period 0 - 24 months Reflex stage	Basic trust vs. basic mistrust—first year Normal symbiotic phase—does not differentiate between self and mother
	Turns to voice and bell consistently Laughs, squeals Responsive vocalization Blows bubbles, "raspberries"	"Circular reaction" the interesting result of an action motivates its repetition	"Lap baby," developing a sense of basic trust
...ween familiar ...ger ...d object ...ror image	Uses single and double consonant-vowel combinations		At 5 months begin to differentiate between mother and self, i.e., beginning of separation individuation Has a sense of belonging to a central person
...y movement	Shouts for attention Imitates speech sounds Waves "bye-bye" Uses "mama" and "dada" with meaning Inhibits behavior to "no"	Can retrieve an object hidden in his view	Practicing phase of separation—individuation, practices initiating separations "Love affair with the world"
...overpronation ...nt	Uses single words Understands simple commands	Differentiates available behavior patterns for new ends, e.g., pulls rug on which is a toy	Rapprochement phase of separation— individuation; ambivalent behavior to mother Stage of autonomy vs. shame and doubt (1-3 yr) Issue of holding on and letting go Pleasure in controlling muscles and sphincters
...rk ...neatly	Points to named body part Identifies one picture Says "no" Jargons	Capable of "insight," i.e., solving a problem by mental combinations, not physical groping	
...ng knob ...ottle or spoon ...ually begins	Two-word phrases are common Uses verbs Refers to self by name Uses "me," "mine" Follows simple directions	Preoperational period (2-7 yr)—able to evoke an object or event not present Object permanence established Comprehends symbols	

Age	Gross Motor	Fine Motor-Adaptive	Personal/Social
3 yr	Runs well Pedals tricycle Broad jumps Walks up stairs alternating feet	Imitates three-cube bridge Copies circle Uses overhand throw with anterioposterior arm and trunk motion Catches with extended arms hugging against body	Most children toilet trained day and night Pours from pitcher Unbuttons; washes and dries hands and face Parallel play Can take turns Can be reasoned with
4 yr	Walks down stairs alternating feet Hops on one foot Plantar arches developing Sits up from supine position without rotating	Handles a pencil by finger and wrist action, like adults Copies a cross Draws a frog-like person with head and extremities Throws underhand Cuts with scissors	Cooperative play-sharing and interacting Imaginative make-believe play Dresses and undresses with supervision distinguishing front and back of clothing and buttoning Does simple errands outside of home
5 yr	Skips; tiptoes Balances 10 sec on each foot	Hand dominance is expected Draws man with head, body and extremities Throws with diagonal arm and body rotation Catches with hands	Creative play Competitive team play Uses fork for stabbing food Is self-sufficient in toileting Dresses without supervision except tying shoe laces Brushes teeth
6 yr	Rides bicycle Roller skates	Prints alphabet; letter reversals still acceptable Mature catch and throw of ball	Teacher is an important authority to child Uses fork appropriately Uses knife for spreading Ties shoelaces Plays table games
7 yr	Continuing refinement of skills		Eats with fork and knife Combs hair Is responsible for grooming

Table from Molnar GE, editor. Pediatric rehabilitation, 2nd ed. Philadelphia: Williams & Wilkins; 1992 Reprinted with permission

Index

W

Tables

Illustrations

The Rehabilitation of People
with Spinal Cord Injury

Shanker Nesathurai, MD, FRCP(C)
Editor

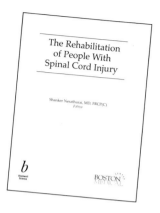

A rehabilitation physician faces no greater challenge than coordinating the
care of a patient with a spinal cord injury (SCI). To achieve optimal outcomes,
the practitioner must understand both the biological and sociomedical issues
associated with SCI. The Rehabilitation of People with Spinal Cord Injury provides an overview of the clinical issues for resident physicians. Other members of the health-care team—physicians, nurses, therapists, social workers—
may also find this monograph of interest as a guide to help them treat their
patients. There are chapters on autonomic dysfunction, bowel care, bladder
function, sexuality, environmental adaptations, and community reintegration,
as well as 20 illustrations.

To Order: Please visit www.bumc.bu.edu/rehab
           www.blacksci.co.uk/usa or contact:
           (800)-215-1000 or 781-388-8250;
           fax orders: 781-388-8270

Other books to be published in this series include:
           The Diagnosis and Management of Bowel and Bladder Dysfunction
           Fundamentals of Electrodiagnosis
           Outpatient Rehabilitation Medicine

Essentials of
Inpatient Rehabilitation

Shanker Nesathurai, MD, FRCP(C)
David Blaustein, MD
Editors

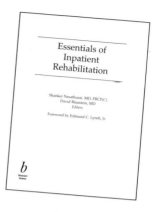

The Essentials of Inpatient Rehabilitation is a concise monograph that reviews the major clinical entities managed in an acute rehabilitation venue. Topics that are covered include total joint replacement, fracture, stroke, multiple sclerosis, amputation, and peripheral vascular disease. There is a discussion of fundamental concepts such as the organization of rehabilitation programs, indications for therapeutic exercise, and the rationale for passive interventions. This monograph contains 142 pages of text and 18 original illustrations.

To Order: Please visit www.bumc.bu.edu/rehab
www.blacksci.co.uk/usa or contact:
(800)-215-1000 or 781-388-8250;
fax orders: 781-388-8270

Other books to be published in this series include:
The Diagnosis and Management of Bowel and Bladder Dysfunction
Fundamentals of Electrodiagnosis
Outpatient Rehabilitation Medicine